DEDICATION

Compromising who you are is different than compromising with someone who is important to you. So, to every man and woman whose heart hurts, and especially if you feel broken, it's not necessarily bad, you just have new choices! Don't give up on love and don't give up on you! ~ Jo Lena Johnson

If you ever felt alone or you ever felt taken advantage of, or you just simply were not sure of your worth in a relationship, I'd like for you to take the time to learn what's important to you. Believe in love and believe in your heart and believe in the truth. Because no matter how hard an individual or situation may try to hood wink you or lead you astray, just remember your friends, your family and God will always lead you where you need to be. ~ Steven Charles Martin

A wise man once said, "The earth has music for those who listen." Listen to your heart and find your music. You can't make someone else happy if there's no joy in your heart. In the end, you must be true to yourself. Find your joy, enjoy your music, live and love. ~ Kevin B. Fleming

COMPILATION

COMPILATION

WARNING

If you are satisfied with your relationship(s) and life,

DO NOT READ THIS BOOK!

Changes in your thoughts may alter your perception.
Things are not often what they seem.
Moving forward – It's Your Choice!

PRELUDE

A MUSICAL CONCERTO
FROM SOUL, ICE AND WATER

Music is the Soundtrack of Our Lives

Think of this book and its musical references as a stage play to celebrate your past, enjoy your present, and change your experiences by strategically planning to enjoy your future as you consider the content and the context of the words and the music...have you had enough war? I'd rather be a lover, and no longer a fighter. What about you?

~ Steven Charles Martin, Ice

One of my all-time favorite songs is "I Need Love," by LL Cool J. It delighted and inspired millions of girls, now women, my age. I appreciate it because it taught me that guys really can and do love. All of us need love, and with prayer, time, patience, tenacity, self-checking, maturity, and willingness to communicate, we each can have the love we need; did I mention prayer???

~ Jo Lena Johnson, Water

We all know and love music. We have songs embedded in our minds which lifted us up or broke us down — depending on which stage of our relationship we were in. In the beginning! Our first dance, our first kiss... but OH! After the love is gone. Can you stand the rain? A house is not a home. That joy turns to pain... Let the rhythm get into you. You can have the greatest love of all.

~ Kevin Fleming, Soul

Woman + Man + Music = Powerful Combination!

Defining Love & War

"On the Wings of Love" Jeffrey Osborne
"I Get So Lonely" Janet Jackson
"War, What is it Good For?" War
"Kung Fu Fighting" Carl Douglas
"Love After War" Robin Thicke

Love – The outpouring of Spirit.

transitive verb

1: to hold dear: cherish.

2a: to feel a lover's passion, devotion, or tenderness for. **b** (1): caress (2): to fondle amorously (3): to copulate with. **3:** to like or desire actively: take pleasure in. **4:** to thrive in.

intransitive verb: to feel affection or experience desire

War

noun [G., to perplex, embroil, disturb. The primary sense of the root is to strive, struggle, urge, drive, or to turn, to twist.]

1: to be in active or vigorous conflict

Definitions from Merriam-Webster.com/dictionary
© 2011 Merriam-Webster, Incorporated

Love or War?

"It's a Thin Line Between Love & Hate" The Pretenders
"Power of Love" Luther Vandross
"At Last" Etta James
"Hang on to Your Love" Sade
"Lately" Stevie Wonder
"992 Arguments" The O'Jays

Let's face it, "good" relationships are some of our greatest desires and "bad" relationships create some of our worst nightmares. Whether you typically read books or not, we all need help – if we are going to stop acting up and end the war that engulfs our lives, strangles the breath from our bodies, and attacks our hearts regularly. Creating loving relationships takes work, intention, and strategy; and that's what you'll get as you are entertained, informed, and turn these pages.

We see you sharing your thoughts and reactions at house parties, around water coolers, in salons and barbershops, and with your friends, male and female, in person, and listening to your favorite DJ stirring you up with the words and the songs that will inspire you.

Tina Turner asked, *"What's Love Got to Do with It?"* Well, a whole lot is our answer. George Benson and Whitney Houston said, "Learning to love yourself is the greatest love of all." Remember that as you consider your choices and pick your battles.

If you are tired of getting what you've always gotten, stop the insanity! Pull off the scabs, let down your guard and open your heart to *Relationships and Adult Conversations*, which will soothe you, quench your thirst, help you cool out, and find your groove.

6

Heartache and Healing from H_2O

"Angel" Anita Baker
"Too Much, Too Little, Too Late" Johnnie Mathis & Deniece Williams
"Nothing but Heartaches" The Supremes
"Lady Love" Lou Rawls
"One in a Million" Larry Graham
"Tell Me if You Still Care" S.O.S. Band
"I Need Love" LL Cool J

The good news about being broken is that it allows God to pick up the pieces, strengthen, bind, and build you up fresh and new, if you are willing to surrender to your future and let Him do it.

I've been in battle, without my armour because I've been operating on a conditional basis. Giving Him things to deal with and keeping the things I wanted. Justifying, reasoning, and rationalizing that everything would be okay. Basically, doing the same stuff I've always done, just in another package.

This book was born out of conversations between my guy, Steven Charles Martin and me. We referred to ourselves as Ice and Water. (He, being made up of the same properties that compliment my own, adding refreshment but not changing me; us melding together and blending.) It was a cute concept and writing a book together was a way to address several issues.

People need practical help with their relationships and too many are suffering; we are a couple in a serious relationship, we like to help people and have some experience (engagements, marriages, divorces, work with people) and good info to share; I needed a way to reach a broader range of people and my previous books, trainings and offerings were virtually unknown to those I am meant to serve; he was beginning to transition into a new phase of his career, wanted and deserved to share his talents with others and I thought it could help him and us; and finally, we would tour the country and the world as "IceWater," filling stadiums of people presenting, teaching and showing people how to be successful in relationships!

Sounds great, right? I did it again! I pushed and pulled. Full of bright ideas, I of my little self started another project that I was driving – not that God was leading. Well, it didn't work the way I planned and here I am; writing this paragraph alone.

Un-Armoured

In the end, my internal battles along with fervent crying out when it didn't feel good, led me to the point where I had to face my own relationship reality:

We were not suited for one another.

This is deeper than it sounds. Ephesians 6:11 says, "Put on the whole armour of God..." What I real-eyes in this moment is that without His armour every one of my relationships is destined for failure – and I know that to be true.

IceWater's cornerstones as individuals were not in place at the time we came together, and though we became a dynamic couple, we were not equipped with our armour therefore; we were not properly suited for one another.

Exhaustion

Internal battles from childhood, past experiences, material realities and current perspectives exhaust us and vaporize people. In an enclosed environment the fumes cause clouds and kill us because we cannot see, let alone breathe.

Caught in the safety of routine, the idea of partnership and the realities of sex, it's natural to fight to stay in the situation. Eventually though, the war ends because either the toxicity consumes; or you or your partner suffocates and figuratively dies.

Desire and Desperation

God is a trip though because He knows my heart and my true desires. So as many times as I get to the brink of my own death in relationships, He keeps rescuing me from complete annihilation because He knows I really want (and need) MY husband (not just any husband) – deeply, truly, and desperately. Yes, I said it – desperately.

And when man finds a wife, he finds a good thing. Being a wife to my husband is part of my destiny.

I can honestly say that I love God more than anything. And He knows it. I know that God is warm and loving and finds pleasure in helping me (and you), especially when we are dazed and confused. Direction is essential in the desire and desperation equation.

I have been embarrassed and ashamed because I have chosen incorrectly, so many times. What I mean is, I've been hardheaded, abrasive, difficult and not focused on priorities so, by the time I get too low, I actually let go enough to reach for Him. Did I mention that I have control issues?

Ice is a Good Guy

With Ice I found a friend, a good teddy bear of a man who loved me enough to see through my talents, faults, and challenges. He stayed with me long enough to be honest with me about things I had been in denial about for years. I love him for that, and much more.

To have someone believe in you is a special thing because there are days when I didn't believe I could do something, or I needed a voice of reason, or heck, just companionship in this world we live in today.

Pressures mount, debts pile, interest compounds yet, in the end, what do we really have but our relationships? Jacked up or not. Finances or lack of them (along with credit, work, etc.), and the way one handles them, impacts our options and choices in the future.

This is true for previous marriages, children, divorces, and behavioral habits like short-tempers, being a work-a-holic, or staying in a relationship until something "better" comes along.

New Experiences

As a single woman with no children, I too, want to give and share love. It feels like it's been bottled up and that sense of longing and belonging is real for me. To see him smile, to hear him be delighted, to yearn to please him, and to receive these in return, soothed my soul and calmed me.

The song says "To love and be loved in return," is one of the greatest things on earth. For a time, we were in it deep. His love, caring, and support built my confidence and brought out the best in me; and I believe I did the same for him.

That's a twofold sword though…I'm not sure if my issues got too big, or I relied on him more than I was trusting in my faith, but we couldn't go on in the same manner. If we don't hold our mate and ourselves to certain standards, it's easy to slip away.

He started distancing himself and I'm not sure if it was his own concerns solely or if it was his soul saying, "something's" not right, like my spirit was telling me.

I Can't Tell You His Perspective

I just know that I needed him to bring some structure to my life because "Single Woman Syndrome" is not becoming. Yet, I also needed more flexibility, less stubbornness, and more generosity from him. Those times when I was getting on his nerves caused him to act "a way" with me and it hurt because I needed love in the place of distance.

I just didn't know how to reach him sometimes. And then it became, "Am I in this by myself?" "Is he giving up on us?" I mean we talked but I wasn't feeling his heart singing to me at times when "I wanted it."

It's funny though because two of his nicknames are "Big Baby and Debo." Oh, you don't know "Debo" the "big bully?" Well in the movie "Friday" he terrorized the neighborhood with his physical strength, taking anything and everything he wanted, with no regard for others. Yet the Big Baby persona is real too.

And the hilarious part is that we BOTH act like those two at times. So, together, in many ways, we make a good combination. Yep, you can tell I still love him. I'm kicking myself for what I keep doing wrong and as I say that, we get to the heart of love.

God's Will, Not Jo's Show

You see, He has saved my life more times than I want to admit. I feel that sick feeling in my stomach as I write this...

My relationship before Ice was a complete and total mess – and the three before that too. The last two situations I was in before him almost took me out – for real, and as you get older, it's hard to re-cover.

The difference during the time of IceWater is that I learned to keep saying, "Father, whatever is Your will for this relationship." And believe it or not, I actually, genuinely meant it, this time!

Internally and externally certain things weren't lined up. Namely, I had lost control over every aspect of my life. I was not in the condition or position to receive this wonderful, handsome, charming, and loving man who, in the beginning, like no other, turned me on in every way.

So, once we started to write this book we covered subjects, created catchy phrases, and also started facing some realities – we had problems. Coming to the surface and boiling over, there came a day when we had to make the best choice for us – be separate or stay together.

As individuals, we both had battle scars, bad habits, mean streaks, self-absorbed tendencies, heartaches, and blind spots, all shrouded in blankets of fear. So, the blankets are not suited for us.

I needed to hear and feel, "I love you, I need you, I'm not going anywhere, you're the one for me, I'm willing to try some of the things you're asking of me, and we'll be okay."

Yep, that's what I needed, right or wrong.

I could pretend I know what he needed to hear and feel but I can't do it. It's his to share. What I can say is that with open communication, patience, and listening, I still believe it's possible to work things out with those you love.

Men and Women

We are different. Dr. Sir Walter Mack said, "Men are like light switches and women are like spaghetti." I laughed at this and as he discussed it during a talk on his book, "*Making Wrong Relationships Right*," it made so much sense!

When a man is at work, watching a game or packing for a trip, he's focused and doesn't want to deal with other stuff – or maybe he can't deal with other stuff and keep his concentration.

Women, on the other hand, we're all over the place like the sauce and the noodles and if we don't have all of the elements – like his input, warm hugs, or assurance then we boil over and can create a mess.

Men, when women reach out, we need to know that you are with us and we'll get through it. Women, when your man shuts down, work to help him be comfortable to open up.

It takes both parties to move out of their comfort zones for the greater good – love. War sometimes ensues because nobody really WANTS to change, stretch, or lose by being humble and admitting defeat.

It's true that women would sometimes do well not to insist to talk about every little thing. It's also true that when women allow men to NOT talk, open up, share, then he may never express what he's really feeling, or simply may not know how to share it.

Don't wait too long because too much distance can open up a crack in Pandora's box and then it could be an unnecessary end because the number one *cause* of conflict is lack of/or miscommunication. Failed expectations are the *source* of most conflict.

Clearly, if any one person or couple had all the answers, there would be harmony on all of earth.

Self-Awareness

We want to be with someone we can trust – but, if I can't trust me, I can't be trustworthy for someone else. So, out of control has meant broken-ness and hopefully, by the time you complete this book, it will mean cleansing, healing, redemption, renewal, and real love.

Moving Forward

What's next? I have absolutely no idea! It's a scary place and a better place because I'm not struggling for control right now. I do battle with my emotions though – so I'm enrolled in the "Create in me a clean heart, restore in me a right spirit" boot camp right now!

Formally and informally, this book could not exist without Steven in my life. I thank him for the opportunity to be with him. I'm not sure what stance he'll take from this point forward, but if you haven't met him yet, you're missing a treasure.

Are You Ready to Get Real?

Money, sex, danger, hurt, healing, and life issues of all kinds are addressed in this book. We cover things that people won't talk about and that's why we struggle; because somebody won't admit that they have messed up, that they are afraid, unfulfilled, or simply don't know what to do next.

Enjoy the musical selections too! Kevin Fleming was my boss when he was Program Director of one of L.A.'s best radio stations, KACE. He taught me a lot about communication, especially when it comes to listening and speaking to men. A wonderful man, a radio industry icon, and an excellent music arranger, Kevin is one of my favorite people and I credit him with much of my past successes. When I wanted to add music to this idea (before it evolved into this book), I immediately thought of Kevin and his lifelong works. So it was a perfect fit; hence adding "Soul" to this experience. Kevin's musical selections run parallel to the words that Ice and Water, share. His choice of songs will help you, make you laugh at times and be fun to look up, download, and listen to during your journey.

Please use what you read as a starting point for your own self-reflection and then to help you and those you love, in relationships.

Though I haven't mastered any of this, starting with self-love to understand that you matter, will help you appreciate and embrace the divine love that God has for you.

That's important because my life-long lesson has been that if I don't take care of myself, I have no capacity to take care of others. The little things like cooking meals for myself, cleaning up the house when I'm not expecting company, spending time meditating, exercising, and simply appreciating being alive are things that I have not done well in the past. Please don't make my mistakes.

There are people, especially women, who will relate to that last paragraph, you are not alone and yes, there is hope and help for you. If you don't relate to it, don't worry, there's something here for everyone, because we are all alive in today's world. In the words of Betty Wright, "No Pain, No Gain." *Together we rise, connected we stand, and in loving relationships, we all win!* ~ *Water*

LIFE

THINGS HAPPEN IN LIFE.

How you deal with those things can make or break you and your relationships. You can ease stress and strain by managing the things in your control and releasing those that aren't.

How's This for Love?

"Lady in My Life" Michael Jackson
"I Can Be Your Hero" Enrique Iglesias
"Saving All My Love for You" Whitney Houston
"Kiss from a Rose" Seal
"Love is a House" Force MDs

"I met Terry in April 1995 while meeting with our pastor for assisting with our church's youth department. In June, he invited me to dinner at his home and had his friends act as chaperones so that I would feel more comfortable. We speed to August when he asked me to marry him (during alter call prayer at church) for which I just shook my head yes. Ten weeks later, we're saying our "I Do's" and we'll be celebrating 16 years of marriage this coming November. Talk about a marriage that truly was blessed by God."
~ *Penny L. E.*

Notice that when this couple met they were actively involved in an activity that they both enjoyed. In this case, it was in the church; and that commonality, coupled with similar beliefs, created a natural attraction.

Most relationships need time to grow so do what you and your partner need to create understanding and build comfort. The Edmonds were not there "looking for love," they were there growing, serving, and giving of themselves. Meeting in the manner they did and getting married so quickly worked for them.

Be encouraged!

Snoring, Emissions, and Body Odor

"Too Funky in Here" James Brown
"Get on the Good Foot" James Brown
"Why You Getting Funky on Me" Today
"Funky Stuff" Kool & the Gang

"Ladies, you may be used to a man letting loose gas, however, whether you are in a marriage, a long lasting relationship, or an overnight booty call, never get so comfortable that you think it's okay to release gas in front of a man. It is not sexy and simply, it's just downright unattractive." ~ Ice

Sure it's not comfortable to talk about, and it's not comfortable to hear or smell it, for that matter. However, when considering being in adult relationships, be sure that you can handle all that comes with it.

Snoring. Light sleepers and snoring don't really mix. Lack of rest and sleep, over the long haul will undermine your health, your mood, and your disposition. Keep it in mind when you choose a mate.

Noxious Emissions. Have you ever been in a deep sleep and all of a sudden you felt like you just walked into a cloud of sewage – or worse? Well, you might not want to admit it, but who hasn't woken up to your partner's bad gas? If you've been spared to date, kudos for you!

Smelly Feet. Yuck. As people age – especially men, this can be a problem. Throw away the old shoes, use odor eaters, get pedicures (yes, you!) and clean your feet – in between your toes, regularly. Soaking feet in a combination of ¾ cup of mouthwash and ¼ cup of hot water is a highly recommended old home remedy known to detoxify smelly feet. The world thanks you in advance for it!

Bathroom Breaks. How funky are you? Everyone needs to go. If you have a small home, apartment, or if you have only one bathroom, there will be times when "it gets a little funky." Make some choices to spare yourself and your partner the embarrassment and the affect of your disposal. Keeping sprays and such in the bathroom helps.

Body Odor. Every body has a scent. Are you attracted to or repelled by your partner's scent? Think about it if you are serious about a real future. Good hygiene habits like regular showers, brushing teeth at least twice a day, washing hands after every trip to the bathroom, and the use of mouthwash, body creams and colognes all help.

"Perfume camouflage... although you may think you hardly sweat, or that you do not exude body odor, if you are doing physical activities there is some type of funk. Don't just come in, wipe off, and spray perfume to cover up the funk. That should never be a woman's choice." ~ Ice

"That applies to cologne too, guys!" ~ Water

Personal Care Works

"Ladies and gentlemen, it's very important to be mindful of your partner's desires and needs. Remember to keep things simple and always try to be pleasing to the eye. Let's not get so comfortable or so caught up with work, caring for kids, or just everyday problems that you do not take the time out to exercise, eat right, and love right. Loving yourself, looking in the mirror, and loving what you

see is the starting point for a nurturing and satisfying physical relationship." ~ *Ice*

Proper diet can make a difference with all of these issues – if you or your partner is willing to take action and change what's not working. Proper servings of fruit, vegetables, and healthy portions can and will make a difference when it comes to weight and the above issues.

But, if there is a problem, the way you communicate needs to be delicate, empowering, and meant to be loving and kind. Don't say, "You stink!" Ouch. At the same time, don't think (and know), "You stink!" and not help them do something about it.

If you notice odors, so do others. It's not fair to you or your partner if you choose not to have the discussion.

Bad Breath and Tough Decisions

"Breathe Again" Toni Braxton
"Hard to Breathe" Anthony Hamilton
"Lose My Breath" Beyonce
"How Do I Breathe" Mario
"Smiling Faces" Undisputed Truth
"On Your Face" Earth, Wind & Fire
How Do You Say What You Really Mean?

One woman put it this way...

My guy worked hard. Standing on his feet, speaking with people, and talking all day, he developed halitosis... this might have had to do with working 14 hours a day, in the hot sun, drinking little water, and having a dry mouth while trying not to go to the bathroom in public places, and holding everything in to get the next sale... I loved him, but the problem got worse and I had trouble being intimate with him.

*I agonized daily because I knew that he was talking with people. His breath was so offensive that customers just had to say "no thanks," because they would not want to smell it. I loved him and was not only embarrassed because of the problem but also for him... hard worker, good guy, prideful and oh, so stubborn... I **knew** his friends had to know... yet people didn't **say** anything... they just avoided talking too long/too close to him... I wanted people to respect him, to **want** to hear the great things he had to say, to interact with him.*

Eventually, we discussed it, and it got better – just a little bit... but not really. Without getting into the rest of the story, we broke up.

I learned a big lesson – that took eight years and a thick skull to get... if there is a problem, it'll stay a problem... if the spark is there, it is. If the spark is not there, it isn't. I could love him yet not want to kiss him because of my flashbacks. Later, when I met someone with a similar problem, I knew that after years in the other situation it would be tough to relive something similar so, I didn't start dating him.

I know I have some ways... that's why I chew gum a lot, don't like people to kiss my ears (I think I can never get them clean enough), and I like to do adult things after a shower for maximum freshness because I would never want my partner to smell something uncomfortable and be too embarrassed to say something to me. I've become very self-conscious by experience.

I should have handled things differently, early in our relationship. I just didn't know what to say or do. I also know that to desire something, one must be that something in order to really get it.

Some things are just tough to talk about. It might seem easier just to avoid but that's not true. Here are some tips for you if you are willing to be courageous and risk a big battle to win the war. If it seems like too much trouble for you to read and consider, maybe it's you, not your partner who really has an issue – we're just saying!

STRATEGIC OPENING LINES FOR INTRODUCING ADULT CONVERSATIONS

Before saying anything, *practice before speaking* to your mate or potential partner. Also, communicating in person would be the most effective if you can arrange it. Think about the outcome you want, and then be prepared to ask for it. For example, ask yourself, "What's the point of mentioning poor hygiene habits or too much foul language in public?"

More than likely, what you want is more frequent showers, baths, teeth brushing, or washing/changing of clothes – because they'll feel better and so will you. Or, it's letting them know that what they say is a reflection of what's in their minds and of their character, and that people judge us by what they see and hear. Since you want everyone who meets them to get the best of who they are, making a slight change in word choice would be a great start.

In cases like these, you want a behavior change. You want the person to do something differently than they have been doing. So, remember that's your goal. Not to complain, put down, nag, or express your disgust or disdain. You want a behavior change.

1. Give a **sincere** compliment/feeling about them. Choose something that is true. Think about their attributes like loyalty, hard working, sweet, smart, or even loving. Examples:

    a. *"You are a wonderful spouse/mate/partner/friend and my life is better because you're in it."*

    b. *"Thank you for your love and support. Being with you is one of the best things that has happened to me."*

    c. *"You have a kind heart and a wonderful spirit. Thanks for sharing them with me."*

2. Then **acknowledge** that the next few things you want to share are not easy but you feel they are important. Saying something like:

    a. *"This is really tough for me to share however, I really care about you, and about us so, would you be willing to listen?"*

b. *"I'm really pleased/happy to be in a relationship with you. I love you and I want the best for you and for us. I've noticed some things over the past few weeks/months and I was hoping we could talk about them and work on it together. Would you be willing to listen?"*

3. Next, **be caring in your delivery** (watch your tone of voice) and also **clear about the issue**. Now that you have their consent, permission to share, and agreement to listen, it should relieve a bit of the pressure. Then go for it.

    a. *"I've noticed that you often leave your clothes in the middle of the floor when you take them off...when that happens, it makes me feel like I'm your maid versus your woman...Would you be willing to put them in the hamper whenever you take them off?"*

    b. *"I've noticed that when we go to bed, you often wear those big pajamas, that (dirty?) head scarf, and your comfortable socks...When that happens, it's hard to get close to your soft skin...What would it take for you to wear sexy teddies at least a few times a week?"*

    c. *"I've noticed that when your children come visit for holidays or over the weekends, they rarely speak to me...When that happens, I think it's hard for me to feel included and like we are a real family...Perhaps you haven't noticed it...What would you be willing to do to help us all have better communication?"*

You get the idea. Remember, your goal is to open lines of communication and have a behavior change. This change may be in your perspective as well, because after you make your statements, perhaps your mate will have some things to share also.

Speaking up about personal things can be really tough. Even if you are an outgoing person, it may be difficult to share how you feel without embarrassing the other person or yourself. However, if you really care about the person, and what you have to say is in the best interests of those involved, choosing to speak up will bring peace of mind and maybe peace in the household.

Moustaches and Excess Hair

"Harry Hippy" Bobby Womack
"I Am Not My Hair" India.Arie
"Hair" Larry Graham
"She's Always in My Hair" Prince

"I dated a girl who had hair under her arms and I thought it was gross and not right. I don't think it's becoming on a woman and it's not the way I was raised. Wearing a dress that shows that, it's just not sexy." ~ Ice

Women, there comes a time when you need to check your upper lip and chin. If it's not quite as smooth or clean as it used to be, take a trip to the salon or local nail shop and get your lip and chin waxed – please. Men, when the hair starts protruding from your nose or ears, please do something about it. Everyone notices it – and it's hard to have the discussion because it's embarrassing for the other person, and probably, especially for your mate.

When chatting about this subject, a friend of ours, KD Washington said, "I'm tired of goatees and breasts." He was speaking about the myriad of women who, as they mature, are not paying attention to the extra hair that is growing.

Be willing to try things like eyebrow waxing or tweezing as well. Neatly groomed eyebrows – not drawn on, too thin or out of control, can and will compliment any face.

Uni-brows – not good for women or men. Enough said.

Just for Men

"Very Special" Debra Laws featuring Ronnie Laws
"Concentrate on You" LTD
"Sensitivity" Ralph Tresvant
"I Thought It Was You" Bell, Biv, DeVoe
"Devotion" Earth, Wind & Fire

"Your time will definitely come, if you can say, 'I am being a good person.' Trying to be positive and doing right by your friends and family, that does make you proud of you. If you can say, 'Yes, I'm doing that,' then you are doing alright." ~ *Soul*

Strategic Planning

Being successful is hard work and it doesn't happen overnight. Through consistent goal setting, positive relations, and fulfilling your strategic plan, success will come. It starts with self. Be proactive, have a spiritual base, fight through adversity, be true to yourself and keep a winning attitude, along with a tenacious mindset (never quit), and be true to yourself.

Things to Do and Remember

1. **Find your passion.**

2. **You must like what you do.** It's hard to be successful if you don't like it.

3. **Be diligent and have "thick skin."** Producing good work is a process of repetition. You must keep asking. You never know when someone will say "yes."

4. **Relax and recharge.** You must stay humble.

5. **Your word must mean something.** Integrity is important, and there's great value in helping people.

6. **Cherish your children.** Children do what you do, not what you say. They will emulate your actions. It's very important to understand and keep that in mind when you have them in your presence…in your life, near or far.

7. **Drugs and alcohol are easy.** There are people who want what they want, but understand that you can't be wide-eyed and open to anything. There are people who will take advantage. That's something you have to learn through experience; it's not really something that people can teach you.

Marriage Can Work in Hollywood…And It Can Work for You, If You Choose to Go That Route

"I've been married 25 years, and I have a very supportive spouse who, not only understands the challenges I face, but tries to help me overcome them. You really need someone who is in your corner, who can see things with a different view, with a different eye; who can check you into reality. That's one of the great things about being married and having a spouse who is not directly involved in the business." ~ Soul

"Mrs. S," who has been married for 45 years to her husband, "Mr. S" says, "We should not try to get things out of people that God did not put in them. Others don't see with the same eyes you do. You can butt your head against the wall, even with yourself. Focus on your talents and gifts and focus on what you do have. Cats don't bark and dogs don't meow."

We agree.

Men and Chores

"Soon As I Get Home" Babyface
"Work to Do" Isley Brothers
"Will Work for Love" Usher
"Workin' Day & Night" Michael Jackson

"If I work all day, come home, and have to pick up dirty socks or clothes left all over the floor, it makes me feel like my man doesn't love or respect me enough to put them in the basket. And to be real, it makes me mad because I feel like I'm raising another child. A hand with things around the house makes me feel good and appreciated." ~ Lady Georgia

A lot of men expect women to be the neat and clean ones. However, men must understand that they too should be clean and neat. Simple things like cleaning off your plate or clearing the table after a meal all helps. A lot of problems at home happen when someone feels like the other isn't pulling their weight or contributing to the household.

"Fellas, it is important to be a partner as well as a leader. In fact, look at chores as a momentum setter as if you were the point guard on a basketball team. This position is key because not only is his job to direct, motivate, pass, and execute all plays from the coach, but he also has to score at any given time. This maximizes the team's ability to consistently flow, and the ultimate goal is achieved." ~ Ice

Men, you really do set the example in the household and no one will question your manhood if you clean the toilet or wash dishes or a load of clothes. If things need to be done, just do them.

Women, When Dealing with Men and Selecting a Mate

"Respect" Aretha Franklin
"Who is He and What is He to You?" Bill Withers
"Who is He and What is He to You?" Meshell Ndegeocello
"Brown Skin" India.Arie
"No Ordinary Love" Sade
"Time Will Reveal" DeBarge

Know and Be Yourself

You must know who you are. Act like a woman — respectable and a valuable, precious child of God who deserves support, encouragement, and good treatment. That sets the foundation for your relationship to another person.

Have and Hold to Goals

Know your goals. Be clear on them and your direction. Stay with them as you meet potential mates.

Don't Express Love Before Receiving a Commitment

Every time that couples share or express love before a commitment, the relationship is poised for sabotage. The woman needs to receive a commitment. This practical and logical expectation is being distorted and misunderstood in today's culture, especially by young women.

Just because a man washes his car, takes a bath, dresses well, and spends $150 on a date, there should be no commitment, obligation, or responsibility on a woman's part owed to a man, because he behaved, the way a gentleman does.

Be Discerning

Practice screening. Women once screened men to see if they qualified for a sound relationship, and if they found that they were not qualified, women said "next" and moved on. Sadly, this is not true now in many instances. Screen the man you meet by asking basic questions when you meet him.

STRATEGIC QUESTIONS TO ASK A POTENTIAL MATE

1. Who are you?
2. What have you done?
3. What have been your associations, experiences, and who has influenced them?
4. What type of relationship do you have with your family?
5. What are your feelings about children now or in the future?
6. Where are you headed?
7. What are you doing now?
8. Do you believe in God?
9. Do you believe in marriage?

These questions, along with behavior that you observe, will help you to discover if he is the type of person who can complement you and help you be your best.

Once you have answers to these questions, and you have seen with your "real eyes," determine if the person is a possible asset or liability.

"Gentlemen, remember you are looking for a mate, an equal partner. We remember the virtues of dining, styling, and profiling but at the same time, every good king deserves a good queen...we as men love to nurture, protect, and provide for our women — and ladies, don't forget that it's a two way street; men enjoy it too." ~ *Ice*

"The Secret Garden (Sweet Seduction Suite)" Barry White, El DeBarge, James Ingram & Al B. Sure

Financial Stability

"We Need Some Money" Chuck Brown
"For the Love of Money" The O'Jays
"Ain't Nothin Going on but the Rent" Gwen Guthrie
"Don't You Want Me Baby" Human League
"Mo Money, Mo Problems" Notorious BIG
"Bills, Bills, Bills" Destiny's Child
"Cream" Wu Tang Clan

Are You Financially Sound?

This is an important question to consider. Technically, it should be added to the **"STRATEGIC QUESTIONS TO ASK A POTENTIAL MATE,"** list as #8 in the previous chapter. However, this issue is larger than just a question. Also, timing and context really make a difference when having money conversations. We didn't want to add it there and risk your going and asking a potential mate this question straight out. If you did that, he or she may take offense, as if you are a gold-digger or something else.

Am I Financially Sound?

This is a question you should ask yourself, because it works both ways. Don't be disillusioned and think that anyone, male or female, will rescue you, nor should you expect that just because a person loves you or appears to be doing well from a materialistic point of view, that all is well at the bank.

Extreme shopping habits have been the ruin of countless partnerships and yours will be no exception if you aren't strategically planning for success. Also, people can be at different income levels so don't have unrealistic expectations thinking that you or your partner will enter in or maintain a 50/50 contribution. It almost never works that way. Your personal habits and what you value are at the core of who you are and how you operate. If your past has not been favorable in money matters, make some new choices and get some new skills if need be.

"I made some poor financial choices, especially in regard to relationships. Some of my biggest decisions were based on 'what I thought we would do together.' Unfortunately, some people just don't care and they will not change because attitudes about money are usually deeply rooted. Especially as you get older it's hard to overcome the realities of money problems and it can also limit your choices of mates. Nobody wants to be 'brought down' by somebody else's bad credit or lack of stability. Some people have a sense of entitlement so, watch that too!" ~ *Water*

"Remember, inspect what you expect and be willing to look at self." ~ *Ice*

STRATEGIC CONSIDERATIONS REGARDING MONEY AND BANKING

1. What do you do with your money?

2. How well do you save money?

3. How well do you spend money?

4. How well do you invest money?

5. Do you typically pay bills on time or are you frequently late?

6. What is your income-to-debt ratio?

7. Do you have a retirement plan?

8. What is your credit score?

9. How do you feel about renting versus home ownership?

10. What is your opinion about how bills and household expenses should be divided?

11. How do you feel about shared and joint banking accounts?

These questions are a good start to finding out if you are fiscally compatible. You must consider for yourself – and then as you get into the relationship, consider other things.

"Financial compatibility is a very important ingredient. It sets the tone on what type of lifestyle you may want or feel you may need. But most importantly, it also sets the tone on what you can both have together and in reality. So, ensure that your financial structure and habits are aligned with the same goals and desires with where you see yourself." ~ Ice

Once you get to a certain stage in life, likely you have had some money problems, set backs, or challenges. It is true that money problems are one of the quickest ways to deteriorate a relationship. It's not just about the money you have in the bank, it's also about what you do with what you have and how much you are willing to work to get what you really want.

Designing a mutually agreeable financial plan and sticking to it, is extremely important for you in your relationship and marriage. If you have had problems in the past, use them as stepping-stones to make better choices in the future. And, even if someone has taken advantage of you before, don't let that stop you from being with the one you love. Just be committed to good stewardship and creating whatever checks and balances you both need to keep everything honest, fair, and in place.

A Love Story

"All I Do" Stevie Wonder
"Any Time, Any Place" Janet Jackson
"He Is" Heather Headly
"Hold on to Your Love" En Vogue
"Love Supreme" Will Downing

We have a story like none other. Ours was a miracle. We met spiritually and then connected in the flesh. Many suitors came forward to declare love to me. However, it was this soul called Tunde that I met through a mutual family friend.

I prayed and prayed for a noble, gentle, soft-spoken, pious man of Islam that took the *deen so seriously that he would bring many believers to include myself to Islam in a most humbling way.

My faith in Islam brought me to a level of understanding. I was submitting my will to Allah, so I allowed myself to be spiritually guided. There was so much support and so much approval from well-wishers, close friends, and most importantly, my mother, who had so much to do with it. Who knows what would have happened if she were not there for me at a moments' call? I love her just so much.

It's quite phenomenal. Most people wouldn't quite understand. I had not met him yet in the flesh. One thing I did know for sure was that it was just right and it felt that way deep within.

From the moment I saw his picture. His eyes told me so. I knew it. HE IS! We started communicating, writing letters, texting, and talking almost six, seven times a day. Oh, how in love is one who keeps each other smiling all the time? We are very much in love.

We were separated because of land and water. He lived overseas, and I lived across the waters. But in all faith our hearts were connected as if we knew each other 32 years ago.

In fact we laugh but we mean it: We often tell each other, we have to spend at least 32 years of our lives together because we missed out. We love each other so much.

When we finally met, we ran to each other full of excitement, looked at each other and when we kissed. I mean when we kissed each other: we were instantly given a kiss of life. Our souls were alive and we were happy.

We didn't know any better than to pull out a prayer mat and pray to Allah. Thanking him for this gift of sincerity and love.

As we walked the streets of Accra and Lagos, many passersby told us we brought back the meaning of Love.

That is how we met!

Mrs. Wen K. A.

*Deen is an important word in Islam. It's similar to saying "the Word" or faith in Christianity.

CHOICES

MAKE INFORMED DECISIONS.

Consider alternatives before doing things that may
have long terms effects on you and
those you care about.

45 Years and Counting

"Sweet Love" Anita Baker
"Now that We Found Love" Heavy D
"Don't Stop 'Til You Get Enough" Michael Jackson
"The Way You Do the Things You Do" The Temptations
"Family Affair" Sly and the Family Stone
"Feel So Real" Steve Arrington

We sat down with a married couple that has shared some "old school wisdom" which has been working for them. No matter where you are, in a relationship or waiting for yours, please consider what they've shared.

Being Together and Making It

"There are two things in life that most people do that they don't have to do, and they should make you happy. They are marriage and having children. No one makes you get married. You do it because it makes you happy. Having kids is not mandatory so when you have kids, it should make you happy. The reason is, those two things that you don't have to do are the two things that could make you unhappy — a problem in marriage or you can't afford kids.

So, what do you suggest?

If you get the proper preparation before hand it will help you. Listen to grown-ups (couples) who have been there and at least consider what they say. Once you marry, it's not about getting another later on. People do it (get married) too soon or don't do it for the right reasons.

If you make it that far, they will eventually be 60 years old, so when you get serious, you have to look at them like at age 60. You have to go deeper than the surface. In other words, don't marry based on surface things that will change.

1. **Be committed.** *Take them and your marriage seriously and honor them.*

2. **Try to find someone you have more in common with than not.** *You don't want to be going in two different directions. You have to have something you can enjoy together.*

3. **Take personal time and develop you.** *The better person you are, the more confident you'll be. Then you're not competing and you'll know your passion. Find your own strengths. Figure out your niche and develop those things in you, and you bring those to the table.*

What about words?

What you perceive as wrong may be based on the way you react or the way you were trained. If other people have conditioned you that certain things aren't right it will affect your relationship.

Math is objective. Words are not and people can interpret in a lot of ways. Two is different than a lot. Words are subjective so don't let words help you jump to conclusions. Words change. Numbers never change.

Be careful with your words and back off with your tone of voice. Sleep on some things, because many times after you think about it, it's not worth it or it's not a big deal.

"If" is a poem by Kipling. Read and think about it. He doesn't let words get to him. It's how you react to things. Listen to the words and don't react. Just keep on going. You don't bark back at the dog or the telephone pole. Especially if (they) are teasing and you ignore them, they'll leave you alone. Dissect it.

What about money and marriage?

As a man I must provide the basics. If that's all we have, at least we are comfortable. If your wife is not working, you should never be in a position that you aren't comfortable. If she's working and you can get more, fine. I never wanted to depend on my wife for the basics. It's icing on the cake, whatever she does. I must make sure I'm prepared for an emergency as a man. As long as you will be warm, eat, sleep, and have a roof over your head, even taking a little vacation, those may be your basics. It ought to be something.

Before I retired, I had a good, solid job and I liked it and then learned to love it. If you are going to be a behind kicker, remember you have a behind and everyone has feet. Do unto others, as you will have others do unto you.

Take care of home first. Make sure your children have what they need, activities, lessons, etc., and have what you need for that purpose first.

What about being "equally" yoked in a material sense?

If you tied up to the wagon pulling with 50 pounds and that's what you had, that's what you had. Sometimes the talk about "equality" has gone too far. There are some advantages and disadvantages to being with a person and everything may not always be there, or may not be what you wish for.

You must make sure there is a commonality. If the person is on the same road and you came from similar environments you are equally yoked. The question is, "Are you both willing to come from the same perspective?"

We should do the right thing because all we've got to do is die. It's only so much wrong you can do." ~ Mr. and Mrs. S.

Real or Representative?

"Can This Be Real?" Natural Four
"To Be Real" Cheryl Lynn
"Real Love" Mary J. Blige
"Real Love" Lakeside
"I'm Real" Jennifer Lopez
"Tell Me It's Real" K-Ci & JoJo
"For Real, For Real" Mariah Carey
"The Real Thing" Jill Scott
"Fake" Alexander O'Neil

Get to Know the Real Person, Not the Representative

In the beginning, nine times out of 10, that person showed you their true self and you dismissed it.

"He was lazy. The only thing he did was go to work. I reared the kids, gave the baths, did the yard work, cleaned the house, painted the basement, took care of the cars, I did it all. Had I known these things before we got married, I would have made different choices.

We couldn't agree on anything – the money or even going to church. He didn't want the kids to go because he didn't want to go. We went on a trip. On our way to the cruise ship, we took two different cabs. It was awful. Things just started to deteriorate and some of it was completely my fault. It's enough blame to spread around, but at the end of the day, we grew apart, really." ~ Mrs. Brumley (Divorced)

About Being Married

1. **Always be true to yourself and know who you are before you try to be married or to be with someone else.** That's hard, especially when you are really young.

43

If you don't, you end up growing apart because the person that you are now is different than the one that they met. You change; it's natural and hopefully, you will both change for the better, and mature. However, relationships grow apart because you are not on the same level or mindset and then things can get out of hand.

2. **Communicate and be honest.** Sometimes that's hard to do. And it's not just men but women have to communicate too. There are questions before and during the relationship that you need to address. If you "change for them" it will only be temporary because in the end, your true self will always win.

   Sometimes honesty is difficult because you don't want to hurt the other person's feelings. However, in some cases, it's that you just don't want to own up to what's really happening because you are getting rewards in some way for staying together; like it or not.

3. **You need to have some commonalties.** The adage opposites attract, that may be true but it won't keep you together.

4. **Have a plan.** Before the marriage, consider things like, "When are we going to have kids?" "Who's going to do the housework?" "What are we planning to do in terms of our careers?" "Do you think we should take a vacation every year?"

These are things you don't think about when you are too busy being in love. These are also the very things that turn around and bite you later because you didn't discuss, weren't honest, or maybe didn't even think about it. The Bible is clear about not being unequally yoked; it's real and it's true.

The idea of marrying for love is great but it is a business agreement. It's a lot more involved than love. We can love each other but that doesn't mean we have to be married.

"Yes, we finally got divorced. I love sleeping in my bed alone – I sleep in the middle. I love it!" ~ *Mrs. Brumley*

"Safe" Sex or Celibacy?

"Sex Therapy" Robin Thicke
"Wishing on a Star" Rose Royce
"Take Your Time (Do it Right)" SOS Band
"You Sure Love to Ball" Marvin Gaye
"Slow Hand" Pointer Sisters
"I Can't Wait" The Impressions
"Anticipation" Bar-Kays

Safe Sex

Safe sex means adopting responsible behaviors when it comes to your sex life. Be willing to talk about it and ask questions. Don't be afraid to confront and address your status, and your partner's status. Discuss issues from birth control to taking rapid HIV tests. Take that next step if you are really grown. If you are in a relationship, you'll know their status; the responsibility is yours in your relationship; you are exposing your partner to everything, including the risk of pregnancy, possibly herpes, and more. Condoms for men and women, as most adults know, will help you. Don't use excuses not to use them, and don't stop using them if you don't have a true, monogamous commitment.

Celibacy

There are many benefits to being celibate. Clarity and ability to focus are two of them. Is your mate or potential mate comfortable with that?

If you are single and you want to have a relationship while remaining celibate, it may not be an easy proposition to pull off. Likely, there will be persons who will lie and say they are "okay with it." But don't mean it or don't take it as seriously as you may.

To those who are mature enough to handle, respect, and deal with this lifestyle choice; don't let someone take you off your course.

Let's face it; expectations in today's world are that people will be sexually active. Celibacy is a personal decision, which will have long lasting effects on your choices of mates and more than likely, on the results of what you ultimately want.

Confidence

"Champion" Kanye West
"The Greatest Love of All" Whitney Houston
"A Woman's Worth" Alicia Keyes
"Let's Hear It for the Boy" Deniece Williams
"Everybody is A Star" Sly and the Family Stone
"You're the Best Thing Yet" Anita Baker
"The Finest" SOS Band

You are Brilliant

Do you know that you were born for a purpose? A big part of your journey is exploring (finding out) and experiencing (living in) your purpose. This can be tough because life happens and it's not easy. Sometimes everyday problems get in the way and then you may act up and start fighting yourself or those who love you.

In those moments when you find that you aren't where you thought you would be, it can rattle even the most determined and tenacious person. Since your accomplishments and your life matter, do what you can and be willing to learn and ask for help or assistance when you don't know what to do. As you grow you will start to share the best of you. Confidence shines through and helps others to feel better about themselves too. So, don't give up!

Confident Men and Women

"Being confident means not being afraid to make decisions, believing in himself, working hard and in his mission to be successful. Though focused, he's not stubborn, and is comfortable asking for directions or help when he's unsure because he knows where he's trying to go. He knows how to be patient and is also

open to trying new things. He can look himself in the mirror and be satisfied with what he sees, knowing at the end of the day that he did all he could to be the best he knew how to be.

A confident woman believes in herself, in her abilities, and in her value. She is comfortable with who she is and with what is important to her. She pays attention to the details about her life, her health, and her passions because that's what a secure confident woman does. In life, be it at home or at work, she often multi-tasks and is independent enough to take charge whenever needed. She is also secure enough to listen, share, and follow the deserving man she trusts." ~ Ice

Insecurities Do Happen

Sometimes in adulthood, people lose their confidence because of past choices, broken relationships, failed careers, or just problems that have happened in life. Whenever "new" situations come up, it's normal to feel uncomfortable so, if you notice that something has come up, just take a breath and acknowledge what's going on.

If you want to be confident, it's important to have a good foundation. Starting with a spiritual connection can often ease fears and concerns and help with self-assurance, clarity, better choices, and loving relationships. Exercising helps also because of the health benefits and let's face it, the visual benefits too.

Help each other out because "That's What Friends Are For," and a key factor of a solid relationship is friendship, coupled with understanding, truth and acceptance. If you notice that your mate is behaving in an insecure manner, turn it into a positive. Take time to encourage them to develop some of their strengths or interests and also help build their confidence with assuring words, open communication, and genuine, loving compliments about things they do well.

STRATEGIC PLANNING FOR LOVE & WAR

Let's Be Real

"They say" that money, sex, and religion are the cause of most problems. We agree that they can create war so, be strategic about how you handle problems.

If weight becomes an issue, get involved together in a health program; don't just expect your partner to go it alone.

Trust Yourself

Relax and trust your partner too. That they want to be with you and are happy with you and what you bring to the table. Make sure you have some hobbies and other interests that keep you occupied – don't let your whole life be your mate.

If you are set in your ways and you won't do anything else, you'll probably end up single. Take your time and listen to all the signals given to you.

Questions, reactions, and the way people behave when you are living your life/work can be affected – patterns arise and you need to have a plan on how to deal with them – if you are going to stay.

Educated women and the corporate workforce are a mixed bag. Meaning that to be successful at work takes certain skills, tenacity, and independence. However, balancing expectations and behaviors in the relationship arena takes awareness, femininity, and flexibility. If women choose a mate who may or may not be college-educated or in the corporate arena, it can cause conflict and tough times in the relationship so, support, good communication, and confidence is needed on both sides.

Consider Your Mate

Women, accept your man and help him feel good about the career he's chosen. Give your man the chance to be who he is…don't be overbearing and remember to come from your heart. Show him the feminine side of you and allow him to love you and treat you like a woman.

"Men, trust your mate and trust that your relationship is strong enough. Strength comes from the heart, it's your 'big' muscle!" ~ *Water*

Improve Your Shortcomings

If you don't know certain things like current events, hot topics or today's issues, an easy way to get informed is by picking up a newspaper or scanning the Internet for news. Just acknowledging what you "know you don't know," by taking initiative to learn more is a great start. You'll feel better and so will your mate.

Whatever attracted her/him to you, the complete you, your health, wealth, and self, keep it up and step it up. Make sure you keep yourself in shape and work hard to be the best in your vocation/career, your fitness, your finances, and work.

Insecure folks will put sugar in your tank, a knife in your tire, mess up somebody's barbeque, and show out in front of others, insecurities with no brakes.

"I Believe I Can Fly" R. Kelly
"I Didn't Know My Own Strength" Whitney Houston
"I Hope You Dance" Lee Ann Womack
"The Greatest Love of All" George Benson

Living Together

"A House Is Not A Home" Luther Vandross
"Home" Stephanie Mills
"I Don't Want to Be Lonely" The Main Ingredient
"Living All Alone" Phyllis Hyman
"I'm Not Your Daddy" Kelly Price & Stokley
"Until You Come Back To Me" Aretha Franklin
"Human Nature" Michael Jackson
"Together" Ohio Players
"After the Love Is Gone" Earth, Wind & Fire
"I Wanna Spend the Night" Bill Withers

Why are you considering living together? How long have you been together? What are your goals for your relationship? Are they the same as your partner's goals?

"Yes, it is my belief that men and women should live together prior to getting married and/or in their engagement stage because that's the true, uncut, down and dirty real assessment of the relationship, the individual and potential path that will be taken from that point (in other words, it's setting the tone for your potential marriage)." ~ Ice

"I think what happens is, living together gives license to put all the eggs in one basket and then one person can come up short, when and if the other person is conditional, i.e. they are not married and they have an out. If the couple isn't ready for real commitment (ultimately, marriage) they probably aren't ready to live together either." ~ Water

In the past both of us have lived with a person with whom we were in a relationship/engaged and it didn't work. We're including this because we want you to know that when you live with someone, everything is exposed. So, it's really your choice – just be ready for what may follow. It could be successful or not – and that too depends on the way you look at it. If you live with someone and see that this is not a person you should marry, and you get out before the vows, that could save you from a lot of heartache in the future, though it will be tough in the short term.

At the same time, the Bible says that men and women are to be married. It's a moral, social, and cultural dilemma that you as an individual need to take seriously. Do what's right for you.

STRATEGIC CONSIDERATIONS WHEN THINKING OF SHARING A HOUSEHOLD

1. What do you really want? Is it financial relief, to be "kept" or to be "kept up?"

2. Control? Of you, the other person, the interior and perimeter of the apartment, home or property?

3. Partnership where each contributes according to his or her ability, resources, and income-to-debt ratio?

4. Really working together is not just about a financial arrangement – it's also about space, freedom to spread out, extending comfort zones, and generosity of time, spirit and closet space. Are you willing?

5. If living together doesn't work out, who will move and where will you live?

When contemplating living arrangements, it's imperative that both parties share in terms of finances, chores, energy/electricity conservation, and also in terms of values.

Common space affords date nights at home with access to board games, playing cards, or a candlelight rendezvous in the kitchen and beyond. Cohabitating allows for companionship, easy-access to shared resources like his pots and her pans; and it also provides an entree to the couples' own haven of safety, love, and security – the ability to tackle the world together.

When considering making a move, think about sharing activities, time, and schedules. Identify the goals of each party as to why you are joining households. No one wants to feel used and everyone has expectations. Be clear on yours and your partner's expectations before jumping into a situation you may regret.

Misery loves company…always remember that because if you share space with it, it will infect and affect you too.

So, What Do You Really Want?

Short term? Long term? For your partner? For yourself? For the relationship? Go in with eyes wide-open and with clear expectations so that you can sleep and rest at night.

Make written agreements, moving condition terms, and back up plans if things don't work out. And create a strategy for maintaining positive attitudes, good habits, and shared responsibilities.

You must be willing to "give up" to receive. Each gets to be understanding, compassionate, and willing to be flexible, loving and generous, including you!

A Cougar's Tales

"Just to Keep Satisfied" Marvin Gaye
"Just in Case" Jaheim
"Just Came Here to Chill" Isley Brothers
"Maybe Your Baby" Stevie Wonder
"Love Makes No Sense" Alexander O'Neil
"Hot Stuff" Donna Summer
"It's Raining Men" The Weather Girls

"It's not the toy itself on the holiday that's the most exciting part, it's unwrapping the package. If you are packaged right, that's half the fun. When my 'boy toy' thinks, 'I wonder and anticipate what you have on underneath — and I get the pleasure of seeing you like that — sexy, mature, and it reminds me of what we see on TV.' It turns me on, keeps me excited, and confirms what I already feel, 'I'm hot!' That's the way cougars roll." ~ Ava

"I tell the young girls when they try to hate or they can't understand and call her "old" she's not old; she's confident, she knows what she wants, she's comfortable with herself, and she's mature; and maybe one day, you can be like that too." Says a man who now considers himself too old to be a cougar boy toy, but enjoyed it before he turned 35 and started being interested in "wifey" material.

"Trust me, cougars do exist; and there are sugar mama's too. They will buy you stuff and all they want is a play toy; someone they can have sex with and then show them off. At 34, I know these women are an option but it's not what I really want." Mr. Jay

How Do You Define Cougar?

Well, Ava, our resident cougar admitted, "I never heard the term until somebody that I was seeing called me that. I think it's when you are having sex with someone when there is a ten year or more age difference."

It's All About Sex

That's what we've been told. Mature women like stamina, a nice sized package and no drama, being catered to in the bedroom, feeling powerful and in charge – getting to call the shots. Variety seems to be the spice of life and smarts are not required.

How many of these young men do you have at any given time?

The most I've had is five. I don't see them all, all the time. Only two are in my city and I'm able to see the others pretty easily.

What are advantages to being a Cougar?

I like being the person in the relationship that knows what to expect and what's to come. I've already been there, I know what they are thinking and there is no mystery with them. In the sense that when you are dating a guy who is age appropriate, you to have worry, "Should I call him?" "Is he married?" "Does he really like me?" "Where is this going?" And in a cougar relationship, I feel like that's what the other person is thinking, not me.

Not having to worry about where the relationship is going is a relief. I already know it's not going anywhere and it's only going to be there as long as I want it – it's just a sexual relationship for me – and then it will be over.

Not having to decide or choose just one makes things easier as well. I can have as many as I want and be honest about it. With young guys I always tell them up front that I'm not trying to marry them, and that I'm not looking for a soul mate. It's easier to be honest about it.

Do you feel this might be perceived as settling?

No, it's the exact opposite. If I were going to settle I would just be with someone my age and call it a day. I think settling means you are coming to terms with what you have and thinking that this is as good as it's going to get. There is no settling with a young guy — they are so eager to please you. They are working so hard to make you happy. They go out of their way to make sure you won't get bored or tired of them. They go out of their way to give you what you want. I think it's because they still have hope for their future, unlike people in let's say their 40s or older. They still think things can happen in their life in their 20s. They are not going to be as eager to please when they are 40. They will end up feeling like they are the gift no matter how messed up their attitude or situation is by then. But in their 20s they feel like they have a lot to learn and they go out of their way to be memorable and such.

You've talked about the relationship aspect; let's get down to the sex.

With the young ones, the door isn't even closed before we get started. Sex is amazing; they don't get tired and their recovery time is like five minutes! Without the blue pill! They are eager to please and that turns me all the way on. It's disappointing with older men in so many ways. I used to think it would be lingerie and candles all the time, however, it's a special occasion like Valentine's Day or his birthday when the woman gets to have her moment when she's with older guys or in a relationship. I don't know what great sex means anymore because after you get married the woman doesn't do the lingerie anymore.

I can remember a time when I was with my ex and I wore this lingerie that had the nipple cut out on the bra. When he took off my shirt and saw that my nipples were out, he started laughing at me. He thought it was so funny — I don't know, I guess it was not the norm for us. He acted as if he had never seen lingerie like that before — I was so embarrassed.

All the things I always wanted to do in my bedroom I now do that with the 23 year olds; they think sex with all 40 year old women is lingerie and candles; and whatever else you hear about in the movies. It's the way you imagine it to be.

And their 20 year old sex partners aren't doing all of this. So the down side of that is this – after you have sex with someone in their 20s, they don't ever want to go away. They are having sex with someone who has been doing it for 20 years, I can tell him what to do to me, he can actually do it, he makes me go crazy, and he feels empowered that he can do it.

And you know, it's good because they are working so hard; and after they [ejaculate], they don't collapse and start snoring immediately.

Sex now is about me and for me; it's not about how quick I can get my clothes off. I would have sex when I was in my 20s thinking that something was wrong with me because I didn't have an orgasm; it was just that I wasn't pleased yet. I'm not embarrassed to tell them what I want. It feels good to know what I want.

Every time I get together with them, I wear the lingerie. So if I would try to hook up with them and didn't set that theme with them they would probably think I was mad at them.

Do you have any stories about "age appropriate men" as you call them?

I reconnected with my first boyfriend ever. I've known him since elementary school. He ended up being my first kiss, my first everything. A while back we reconnected on Facebook(R). I had told him that I had only been dating young guys and it was nothing serious. Our feelings ended up reemerging from when we were little. I even felt marriage could be in our immediate future...he has a beautiful, crazy body and his body intimidated me – it looks really good.

We hooked up, music was on, lights were off, I had cooked enough food for days so we didn't have to leave the hotel room. He walked into the room, turned on the light, and picked up the remote. After waiting three hours I began kissing him so we could get started. We did it and the sex was good; I was ready to do it again and he was like, "Don't be mad at me — I need water, cold water, and a little time, for real. I need some rest and down time."

I was ready to get more 15 minutes later and he was like, "What are you doing? I don't have anything else." He said, "I'm going to need some time — 30 minutes…" He started snoring during the time we were talking. I left him alone for about 1½ hours… finally, at midnight he did it with me again — out of sympathy, and reluctantly. He said, "I can't recover that quick I have to have complete down time." So, I left him alone until two or three in the morning, and I was ready to get some more. He said "I don't know what's wrong with you, I am proud of myself, I haven't had sex like this since I was in my 20s but you need some more and I don't know what happened to you…"

This is what being with 20 year olds has done… his body is banging and I didn't understand how he could look so good and be so fit, yet not be able to continue to have sex. He explained, "I have stamina to run and such but that doesn't have anything to do with the stamina of my D; my D is 42 and my D cannot be lied to." I was so pissed at the time; it was 6 am, I wanted more; I didn't understand. He took my hand off his D and pushed it away…

I was thinking, "I gave you six hours between sessions. "What do you mean you have nothing left?"

He showed me that the 42 year old D couldn't do me up the way I was used to being done up, and all that talk of getting back together was out the window. I was no longer remotely interested in being with him anymore.

He wouldn't have sex with me the next day so, I checked out of the hotel and left two days early because I didn't get together to have sex only one time each day. I wasn't mad at him, but I didn't want to stay in that hotel room watching ESPN with him for three days.

He calls me all the time and wants a do over – he thinks he's ready. We don't have to have a do over – we are good.

He thinks I'm destroying the youngsters for the other women.

D.C. Baby!

My young friend in D.C. – we'll be at it for 40 to 45 minutes and he'll have an orgasm really, really hard and not collapse on me. And after he does, he will not stop doing me; he will keep going and then he'll ejaculate again in 15 or 20 minutes.

The first time we got together we had sex like eight times in a 20 hour period; and the last time we had sex he was like, "I think we have a problem – the condom broke; it's empty." I said, "You just don't have any semen left." He didn't believe me and believed the condom was broken. I told him to fill it with water and when he did, he saw that it wasn't broken, and that no water came out.

He said, "Where is the semen?" I said, "Your body hasn't regenerated more semen." He said, "I felt it." Meaning he had the orgasm (but no fluids)... He said, "I never heard of anything like this – you broke my joint!" I told him, "Don't worry, it's not broken, after you rest, you'll get some more." And, of course he did.

He aims to please me and it's a big deal to him that he's with someone who's 40ish. I like the feeling that I'm the expert in the room. D.C. is my favorite. He's appreciative of whatever I do, like when I wear new lingerie. He notices things that you want your man to notice when you are older – even if it's a new pair of panties. I had always wanted to have sex in a limo but it had never

*happened. One day I surprised him and we both had the best time —
he had never been in one before and we went all around the city —
having sex in the back of the limo, in between sightseeing. It was a
fantasy come true in more ways than one, for both of us.*

*Yes, I have sex on my mind. I love having sex with D.C. but I don't
even need to talk to him. He uses terms that I don't understand, he
listens to artists and music I've never heard of…if we are making
plans to see each other or talking about sex it's great. He didn't
even know who a very well known former female candidate was in
2011! He doesn't need to be smart, I'm not trying to keep him or
have a relationship or have kids. When he gets a girlfriend I don't
see him at all; when he's in between, we get together.*

*I don't need to know who she is; and I admit that when she (the
first girlfriend) came on the scene, it bothered me a little bit — but
not that much…he's 28 and we've been having sex for three years.*

*I always know he's not going to be in a relationship long; he's
immature. He's fine, sexy, cute, still lives at home, spends $100 on
sneakers and $40 on hats, talks like a teenager, and hangs out
with his boys…so a 24 or 25 year old is going to stay for just a
little while, thinking he's going to change because she wants to get
serious. If he told me he had a girlfriend who was 40 I would keep
on doing it though. I wouldn't get out of the way for that, but I
would get out of the way for someone who had potential to be his
soulmate.*

I Had a Husband

*I wanted to have sex like this with my husband; I just had the
wrong husband. I asked him to scratch me or bite me or give me a
hickey and he wouldn't do it. He said to me one day, "I have a
mental block and I hate to think of other men ever being with you."
And because I was so good at sex, he was uncomfortable thinking of*

what / who I had been with in the past...he couldn't believe I could give a "mic check" like that (you know, testing, one two, one two).

I learned that if I did it doggie style with him and if he did three pumps he would come so, I started just starting off that way and get it over in five minutes and then go back to whatever — it was my obligation.

Have you always had such a high sex drive?

When I turned 38, it kicked into overdrive. That's when it started for me, when I wanted it all the time. I would see images on TV when someone would be in a hotel room or on a balcony and I would think that would be a perfect place to have sex. I think about sex all the time, however, since I have work and responsibilities, I don't have the time to get together and do it as much as I want.

When a man comes for me, it makes me hornier; so, I'm ready to keep going; and the younger ones make sure they keep going because they assume that by the time they get to 40 that men would still be able to keep going at that time.

My stamina and sex drive is amazing. And I'm out of shape; I'm working to get in shape so I can go a lot longer...I get mine first; I usually don't sleep while I'm with them at the hotel. We'll be there two days and I want to use all of that time to do it.

What about married men?

I don't mess with married men ever. If I'm seeing you, and you tell me that you have a girlfriend, I don't see you. I don't want to be in the position of being a mistress — I can't be bothered with that kind of situation. Like when to call, looking at the time, needing to monitor what texts or pictures I send. So, it's not worth it and I won't be bothered.

Wow! In closing, what else should people know about Cougars?

I don't want to hurt anybody. I definitely need to take care of me right now. It's just supposed to be fun. You're not supposed to marry them.

In the words of St. Louis Songstress Barbara Carr, "*If You Can't Cut the Mustard I Don't Want You Licking Around the Jar.*" Choices!

Long Distance Relationships

"I Hope that We Can Be Together Soon" Harold Melvin and the Blue Notes
"Mr. Telephone Man" New Edition
"International Lover" Prince
"Get Here When You Can" Oleta Adams
"Ain't No Mountain High Enough" Ashford and Simpson

"It's only four hours away. We can see each other every couple of weeks and talk every day. We'll make it work!" ~ Water, Being optimistic

"It's hard." ~ Ice, Being honest

When considering long distance relationships, listen to yourself and your mate. They can work, but it's not easy and may or may not be for you.

Four Main Reasons People Get Together

1. Companionship/Security

2. Love

3. Sex/Ego

4. Financial Stability/Escape

Long distance relationships may not work over time, because if you don't spend regular time with your partner, you aren't there after hard days, bad days, and long days. You're not there to share meals, small talk, or to help with things around the house. The longing for sweet, juicy kisses and the seemingly endless nights of full moons filled with sexual desire and need for creative expression and intimate connection are real.

When lonesomeness sets in and your mate is in another city, it adds a layer of complication because if you do go out for a drink, a meal or to hang out, it's likely that you'll meet people. Namely persons of the opposite sex; and if you're not careful, exchanging numbers leads to calls, dinners, collaboration on little projects around the house, from work or that itch you want scratched in between the sheets.

"I work a lot and for really long stretches of time. Sometimes I just need big hugs and time in the same room. If he doesn't feel the same, and do something about it (get together), I start to withdraw and wonder if we are doing the right thing by trying to maintain a relationship. Sure, the love is there, however without the companionship, at times I question if it's what I really want." ~ Water, Being real

From experience, we've learned that in order to keep things going in a long distance relationship, you and your mate must be honest about the present and the future. If you have a future, someone will need to move (if commitment is your ultimate goal). Being truthful about your needs, desires, faults, activities, and choices is the only way to make it successfully to what you both say you want.

Frequent visits, trust, quality time, varied activities (outside of the bedroom), good listening skills, open communication, acceptable codes of conduct with regard to others, strategic planning for when you will both reside in the same city and how to make that happen, along with phone sex and phone prayer time are what we recommend to help you and your partner stay connected as you explore if long distance is a real option, in the long run for you.

Deal Breakers

"Pain" Ohio Players
"Go Away Little Boy" Marlena Shaw
"Addicted to Love" Robert Palmer
"Why Do Fools Fall in Love?" Diana Ross
"Get Away" Earth, Wind & Fire

"Smokers need not apply. Right or wrong, smoking doesn't work for me and my personal space." ~ Water

Deal breakers can be seen as codes of conduct or standards that an individual consciously or subconsciously chooses. They can be about little preferences like not preferring cigarette smokers or requiring that your mate be an excellent cook or dress a certain way. They can also be based on judgments or experiences from a person's past.

Following your intuition is good – but following a path of past hurt and pain is not. One of the reasons it's so easy to "be at war" is because sometimes our deal breakers don't let us get out of the gate with a person. This can be good or not so good.

You have a right to have pet peeves. Sometimes however, those superficial things like what a person's toes look like or being concerned that they don't have the same level of education may prevent you from having real love with the person meant for you.

When you do consider a relationship, agreeing on what will work for you and what won't is crucial to your success. However, there are also more fundamental issues that you should certainly consider and discuss...

"Going through my phone – that's a no, no."~ Ice

Can You Really Handle the Truth?

Sometimes you get into situations where you think you can handle the everyday problems or baggage that your mate brings to the table. Once you commit to the relationship, it's hard to get out. However, you may be creating war on all fronts if you stay. There are serious consequences when blending habits and families…Battling can take place on every front. War with the child's other parent, the kids, your mate, and your inner self may not be worth it.

Dawn Landrum-Ferguson, a Certified Hypnotist and Life Mastery Mentor, says that the minds of men and women work differently.

"As far as money goes; Men use money to Provide, Protect, and to Gain Power. Women use money to Nurture, Enhance, and to Gain Status. The challenge comes in when either of the sexes uses money to hide from life; men will use money to avoid feeling in relationships, women use money to avoid dealing with relationships."

Watch What You Say and Do

We all know that actions and reactions have consequences. Many uncomfortable situations ignite because of a few words, and they escalate with a few more (Fussing, cussing and name-calling?), along with tone, pitch or possibly volume (Yelling?). How you say things is crucial, and what you say is, as well.

Women – Don't threaten to call the police on your man if you don't mean it. A man needs to know that you won't call the police unless it's truly necessary. Don't threaten to call them – make that the last option because it could be the end of your relationship in more ways than one.

This is not about accepting domestic violence – if there is a volatile situation and you or someone in the home/space is in danger, by all means, seek protection, safety, and help. That being said, sometimes people speak out of turn when they feel hurt, threatened, or angry.

Why? Domestic violence is serious and police are charged to protect the victim. When they come in for domestic violence, they come in to squash, with all speed and they won't walk away until the woman is safe, and more than likely, the man will have to leave his house.

If he can get over the fact that you called the police, he may end the relationship because you called the police on him and he may not deal well with the embarrassment and feeling emasculated.

Men – Don't call a woman the "B" word. That's often a deal breaker for women. Even if she takes you back, she will never forget that you sunk so low as to call her that name and you meant it at the time. And be warned, depending on the type of woman you are dealing with, she may cut you, test you, or plan to leave you because her heart and womanly soul feels broken.

Couples – Don't knowingly mismanage community funds. If you are not good at budgeting, tracking, or spending, let your partner do it. Because if you continue to make the same mistakes, it will hold the relationship back and it will end. It's just that simple.

Sex as Warfare

Don't use sex as a weapon or reward. It will ruin your relationship. Your partner could take it, as being rejected or that you don't care about their needs. And hence you create an environment for someone else to come into your relationship. And now, the person can say, "They forced me to cheat."

Don't Chastise or Have an Argument in Public

Someone may feel the need to act out and it could become physical. Perhaps, they may feel embarrassed and belittled in work environments or in front of friends or families. They won't get over it and they won't forget it. You are testing his manhood and he may feel he can't let it go. The issue you were arguing about may have had merit however, a man's pride may be all he feels he has, and if you take that away, you've driven him away and are now by yourself.

A Love Note

"Betcha She Don't Love You" Evelyn "Champagne" King
"Looking for a New Love" Jody Watley
"Feel Like Makin' Love" Roberta Flack
"Love's Holiday" Earth, Wind & Fire
"Knocks Me off My Feet" Stevie Wonder
"Knocks Me off My Feet" Luther Vandross
"Please Don't Go Away" Marvin Gaye
"Lovin' You" Minnie Riperton

Sometimes you can meet a person and they just turn you on. There's a time of getting to know, enjoying one another, and dating. Then, usually one person wants to get serious and if it is mutual, outstanding! But, what if the desire for commitment isn't mutual? You have some choices to make.

"If you allow a person to put you on their 'B' or 'C' team, they'll get a lot of benefits because their 'A' player/partner gets the 'Star' treatment and you get what's left. If that's okay for you, so be it."
~ Water

There are times when, after you've been hanging out with someone for a while, you need to make some choices for yourself, then allow them to – if you are okay with sharing or being part of a team, don't even read this section...

Territory is a Funny Thing...

You bring out the raw in me and I kind of like it...Expansion. Adventure. Restriction. The old, any room for the new?

Uuhhm, umm, ummm. When we are together I feel good. Real good. I feel fire...the landscape, the territory, the rough terrain. It's full of stuff yet there is so very much to gain.

70

When I think of you…I feel you – and it scares me. I look in your eyes and I know you see me – all of me – my vision, my passion, my warm womanly glow, my fire, and mine and your desire.

When I look at you…you feel me – and it makes me nervous. You look in my eyes and I feel you – the depths of you, the breadth of you – your passion, your fire, your past, your present, and something else – the comfort and need of me – and it scares me.

I want you – inside me, around me, loving me – and you want me – and it's good to be wanted – and good to give and receive – and that too, scares me.

Territory is a funny thing – it limits our choices and complicates our adventure…

They say to love and be loved in return is where it's at, but two cannot occupy the same space and time…

Expansion, a bigger field, fewer rules, and new is what we both need and deserve yet, only one can occupy the same space – it's not big enough for two…

One of me is enough of me – and yet not enough for you…I love you, I enjoy you, and I appreciate you. When and if your territory changes and you are ready to really play let me know because the fire will consume otherwise…

I do feel you. You do feel me. I am the cake and the cherry too. My fire – your desire…what are you going to do?

~ A woman who chose not to stay

SEX

MARRIAGE? ONE NIGHT STANDS? WHIP APPEAL?

Wet, deep, sweet, hard, soft.
Power!

Fire and Desire

"Always & Forever" Heatwave
"Forever, for Always, for Love" Luther Vandross
"Forever, for Always, for Love" Lalah Hathaway
"Whip Appeal" Babyface
"My, My, My" Johnny Gill
"You Want This" Janet Jackson
"Whatever You Want" Tony Toni Tone

"I remember when I used to love them and leave them — use and abuse them…then I laid eyes on you…it was pain before pleasure…"
~ Lyrics from "Fire and Desire," by Rick James & Teena Marie

Sex is not a weapon and it should not be used for punishment or to reward good behavior.

Reformed Player

Remember fellas when you used to wine and dine, style and profile and have women flowing left and right? Start a night with one woman and end the next day with another? At some point the game gets tired and you look to settle down. You look to have that mate that will make you feel like all is forgiven and all will be well. So, just remember you may have it going on right now, but when it's all over, you want Mrs. Right to help slow you down.

"Diva is a level of sophistication and confidence. When you walk it's like you demand attention and your presence is automatically felt. Your presence as a woman is captivating and breathtaking. Sexy is sensual, sophisticated, inviting, passionate, sweet, and a downright diva. That's what I like." ~ Ice

Off the Market

Klymaxx said it, "*The Men All Pause*" and they got it together with "*A Meeting in the Ladies Room.*" Looking across the room, thinking *"Whatta Man"* in the words of Salt-N-Pepa; scoping them out, walking around the dance floor seeing and being seen. It's all part of the game that we play and it starts off early in life, at the school dances, and continues in the clubs.

"Eventually, you just want to cuddle with that man that makes your toes curl and whose chest you can lay on – enjoying all of him, including his words, his actions, and even his scent. He's handy, he's hardworking, he's loving, he's sexy, he's responsible, and when he looks in your eyes, you start to melt. That's what I like." ~ *Water*

It takes an instant to meet your Mr. Right or Mrs. Right, and sometimes years before the both of you realize it…

"777-9311" Morris Day and the Time
"Baby Got Back" Sir Mix-A-Lot
"Strokin'" Clarence Carter
"Now That We Found Love" Heavy D

Freak Factor

"Super Freak" Rick James
"Sexy MF" Prince
"Sexy Back" Justin Timberlake
"Moments in Love" Art of Noise
"The Freaks Come Out At Night" Whodini
"I Want Your Sex" George Michael
"Sweet Sticky Thing" Ohio Players

"Sex with my husband is not great. I've had great. Thank God I have memories!" ~ Mrs. Hunter

The relationship won't go well in terms of fidelity if you don't have similar freak factor levels.

"I had two friends who had been married and gone through a lot of drama with their spouses. After they got divorced, I introduced them and thought they would make a nice couple.

They hung out all the time and from the outside things seemed to be going great. After about six months, all of a sudden he didn't want to see her anymore. It took another two months for me to track him down and find out what happened. He didn't want to tell me and finally after I pushed he said, 'She's a prude. She's like a wet fish in bed. She doesn't want to do anything, not experiment or anything.'" ~ Miss Lydia

When you get in your new relationship, that's not you – that's your representative; that wasn't the real person and he or she was doing what they thought you wanted them to do and vice versa. When you change for others and for society it is usually a disaster in the end. That's why divorce rates and infidelity are so high.

"We had been talking and had been discussing intimacy and he said, 'Would you think less of me if I asked you to pee on me?' He's a jokester and I thought he was kidding but he wasn't. I was like not only no — I was like Hell no!

We didn't pursue a relationship because he had been saying some other borderline stuff and that took us over the top. I was really digging on him and I'm glad we had that conversation because I could have ended up in a serious relationship with him and we would have had problems over that." ~ Miss Cynthia

"As a woman, I enjoy oral sex; giving it and receiving it and I know this. A man I was dating said, 'I ain't eatin' nothing that can get up and walk away.' That was good to know because we could have ended up being together…Even though he did it later, because he did evolve and grow. There are some people who are like that and they aren't going to change. ~ Miss Lydia

People can influence us, we can watch TV and all that, but we are who we are at our core? On a scale of one to 10 how freaky are you?

What is your Freak Factor?

You don't want a one or two with a ten because it will never work. You may start doing something with someone because you like them, but once the newness wears off and you get to the real part of the relationship and the honeymoon is over, you're like "and that stuff you do to me, I really don't like" because again we have gone back to our core.

This is not a formula; it's just an outline to consider…

Level One – Missionary. Pretty much woman on the bottom, man on top; occasionally, and that's pretty much it. You gotta do what you gotta do.

Level Five – You would be freaky with your partner, but you're not down with introducing someone else into the mix.

Level Ten – You are pretty much down with whatever; multiples, anal, orgies, as long as it don't have to do with children and animals, you are pretty much down (or up) for anything that is legal. This probably includes swinging, urinating, choking, performing in front of strangers, and maybe S&M.

Let's be clear – those that do things with children and animals are 10+s and that's a whole nother issue. Enough said.

You must be able to have intimate conversations with your partner – think about it; if you can share your body, but you can't share your deepest thoughts, then there is something wrong.

STRATEGIC FREAK FACTOR DETERMINATION QUESTIONS

1. Do you feel obligated to have sex because that's what your partner expects but you really don't like it?

2. What will you not do? In other words, do you know your boundaries?

3. What are you willing to do?

4. What are you interested in doing?

5. Does it matter who you are with when you are doing it?

6. Do you care about who sees what you are doing or not?

7. Do you fantasize about threesomes, joining the mile high club, or playing as or with a dominatrix?

8. Do you wonder what it would be like to include your friend's spouse in your bedroom – both of them or one of them?

9. Have you ever reached your limits?

10. Are you curious about something and you've wanted to explore it, but haven't figured out how to make that happen (yet)?

11. Have you told your partner or mate what truly turns you on? Maybe it's sex toys, other women, other men, or phone sex?

12. Do you like oral sex? And that's giving, not just receiving?

13. Would you expect me, as your partner to participate in anal sex?

14. Are you open to different aspects and levels of activities? Would you do it outside, go to sex clubs, or perform phone or video sex for or with me?

"Ladies, as you think about the 'Freak Factor Levels' and the strategic consideration questions, understand that somewhere, somehow, you fall in here. I strongly suggest that although sex is not everything; understand that it plays a significant role in a physical relationship. With that being said, please be honest with yourself and also with your mate as to what you can take, what you can give and what you are willing to venture to do." ~ Ice

At the end of the day, or night as you will, you should find someone within a couple of numbers of your freak level to be sure that each will be satiated.

Advice On Sex and Marriage from A Married Man

"Let's Get Lifted" John Legend
"Share My Life" Kem
"Oh Girl" The Chilites
"Ribbon in the Sky" Stevie Wonder
"Spend My Life with You" Eric Benét & Tamia
"On Bended Knee" Boyz II Men
"Can't Get Enough of Your Love Babe" Barry White
"Stay" The Temptations

Sex

If you stay married to the same person for a long time, you're going to have problems with sex.

You see younger women out and you want your wife to satisfy you when you take yourself home. Thinking about the way they would do it, that's a fantasy because you know what you had before you left. It's a bad thing to think that your wife will perform any different than she has been and it's not going to work. Your expectations will be too high.

Your actions have to come from the heart. Keep treating her the way you did when you got her. If you don't, your relationship will suffer. And the opposite is true; a woman needs to treat her man like she did when she got him.

Counseling

If you are dating someone and if they have messed up stuff from the past, they need to get counseling before getting married. If you are already married and you are having problems, get some help.

Men, don't be afraid to go to counseling. If you think you're right then you really have nothing to lose. If you go and you are right, then you will be proved that way. Go to counselors who are husband and wife. If they don't put God first and talk about Christian views, they aren't talking about anything anyway.

If God is not the center, it's not going to ever work. Relationships are not supposed to happen if you aren't married. Fornication and adultery are in the Bible for a reason.

As you mature, don't go looking for someone 20 years younger, you're going backward.

You just can't come to bed and you haven't taken a bath, you have to cut your fingernails and keep them clean, and keep your appearance up.

And when you think about cheating, wrap your arms around the woman who has been there for you. Spend your energy on her and being closer to her. Stick with the one you've got because if you go somewhere else, you'll create more problems. Plus you don't know what you're going to get." ~ *Mr. Dominic*

Mr. Dominic has been married almost half his life now (close to 20 of his 41 years). He admits that he messed up when he was younger but, his wife was "raised well" by her grandmother and somehow she hung in there with him while he matured and became the husband she deserved. He's grateful for his wife and is honored to be her husband.

Threesomes

"Secret Lover" Atlantic Starr
"In Love with Another Man" Jazmine Sullivan
"I Should Have Cheated" Keyshia Cole
"You Me & He" Mtume
"Who Is He?" Bill Withers
"I'm F**kin' You Tonight" R. Kelly
"Contagious" Isley Brothers

Are you in the lifestyle? It's a typical question in big cities like Atlanta where it's a secret way of life for many. For singles, it's like having all the cake and the icing without the commitment – partaking of getting freely freaky. Swinging means you have a "committed" relationship and you invite a third party to have sex with you and your mate.

"Yes, I asked my woman to swing because I wanted to have (a) threesome. It was a sexual fantasy of mine and I wanted to know if I was up to the physical challenge. One of the best things to come out of those encounters was knowing that I was up to satisfying two women at the same time. They loved it. Performing like that was really good for my ego." ~ Mr. Paul

It may be a fantasy and may even be cool, however, before you go down that road, know that the cost of sharing may be more than you are ready to invest.

"People are tired of mundane sexuality and what society places on relationships; I think it's more than just sex. It's an experience of sensuality and stretches the limitations of sexuality. I don't think people can recover easily from it; people want that new feeling. They recognize that sexuality and sensuality are limitless and they are the risk takers and the gamblers. I'm not speaking for all of them but, that's what I think." ~ Lady Kay

While there does seem to be a double standard, as two women with one man seems to be more acceptable, Swinger Clubs do have rooms where two men can get together with one willing woman. And then there are the "special" evenings like bi-nights and dark room nights where everything goes down in the dark.

So, a bi-curious woman wants to explore and "get the best of both worlds?" She and her man agree to "their rules" then she goes in search of a woman of her choice, usually in a social atmosphere with her man within eyeshot, watching the seduction begin. She hunts in search of the "right fit" for them because it's easier for a woman to pick up another woman. It's also less intimidating for the woman to choose the one who will join. This also maximizes her feelings of control and dominance – assuring her that she chose this person, not her man; and the other woman is not seen as a threat. You see, if the man had chosen, she may feel insecure and wonder why he wanted her.

Concerns Work Both Ways

"Afterward, I didn't like wondering if the two females would hook up behind my back, or would they be willing to get with another guy. Not knowing the intentions or motives with each person can be a little unsettling, especially if you are doing "it" with your own mate and then adding a third party to the mix." ~ Mr. Paul

Why Share Your Man with Another Woman?

One young lady puts it this way:

"I did it because I'm freaky, I was bi-curious and he talked me into it. And then it got real ugly from there. It turned into the sex clubs, the dirty beds, and people grabbing at you from every which way. It

was real crazy. He got so addicted that he crossed boundaries that weren't supposed to be crossed. We had agreed to rules and then he did something that he didn't have permission to do...you can't do this particular sexual act with a person; you must wear a condom; don't kiss them, you know, things like that.

If I could go back before the first time we did it, I would say 'No' because it turned him into something I didn't recognize and he hasn't come back from it.

It didn't work out in the end. I look at him in disgust because of what he did and he just wants to keep doing it. He continues to put pressure on me – and I still date him." ~ Lady B.

Yes, two consenting adults can consider every aspect of that lifestyle, as the human body itself is a beautiful thing. Some people believe that you can have feelings for both sexes and have lots of fun being in groups. Yet, when you live a certain lifestyle, you forget what normal is. You can go to a regular party and think that it's a swinger's party if you are so into that; it's like the Twilight Zone. At least, that's what we are told.

"So, even though the physical act was an ego boost, the reality is that I wouldn't marry a woman who does threesomes with me because I don't think the ideal marriage would involve introducing new people into our bed.

Men, I can assure you that it's something that tempts the flesh, satisfies the ego, but it will destroy your trust. So, be careful because you just may get what you think you want." ~ Mr. Paul

STRATEGIC QUESTIONS WHEN CONSIDERING THREESOMES

When you open up your "relationship" to another person, you are taking a risk. If you are initiating doing this, how would you react if your lover reacts more excitedly to the other person than he or she does with you? So, ask yourself these questions before you initiate or consent to a ménage-a-trois:

1. Why do I want to do this?
2. Why would my partner say yes to this?
3. What if one of us likes the other person better?
4. What does the third party want/stand to gain by getting with us?
5. What are the rules?
6. Is this a one-time thing or going to be a habit?
7. Are we going to use protection?
8. Are the risks worth the reward? Why or why not?

Some people get addicted to having threesomes and they may even enjoy being with persons of the same sex, secretly, while pretending that you are all they need and more. Since you're an adult now, know what you're getting into before getting down.

> "Trying to Love Two" William Bell
> "Cheating in the Next Room" ZZ Hill
> "Curious" Midnight Starr
> "Don't Go to Strangers" Chaka Khan
> "I Wish" Carl Thomas
> "Everything I Miss at Home" Cherrelle

Men and Motivation

"You Are" Charlie Wilson
"I Like" Guy
"Let's Get It On" Marvin Gaye
"Let's Groove" Earth, Wind & Fire
"I Like What You're Doing to Me" Young & Company
"I Have Learned to Respect the Power of Love" Stephanie Mills

"At your best, you are love, you're a positive, motivating force within my life." ~ Lyrics from "Let Me Know," Aaliyah

"'I need a woman to motivate me to make a whole lot of money.' When I was in Chong Wah, my favorite St. Louis Chinese food restaurant, and I heard a man say that, I smiled, then chuckled, then thought, I kinda like that! Let me find out more!" ~ Water

Mr. Mac says:

When a woman motivates a man, it affects his mind, his love; it encourages him to go forward and to do things. Together, they are able to motivate one another. If we (they) are put together by God, divinely connected, that right soulmate who makes me laugh and happy, my helpmeet, we can agree and be motivated.

But, in the wrong relationship, when we're arguing, disagreeing, and having problems, how could that motivate me? It cannot.

The man that finds a wife, he finds a good thing and he obtains favor from God. When we are in tune with spirit, that's when the relationship is able to weather the storms and adversities that come up.

If you stop in the day of your adversity you are smaller. But, when you learn how to deal, things go smoother, you grow, and it gets deeper and better. If you don't have that divine Godly connection, you won't be able to adjust. You'll get attitudes and be ready to go to divorce court within six months of the marriage.

When you're in it and it's not of God, and you encounter areas you have information about, and you know that you are unequally yoked, there will be clashes...a lot.

Even when things are really bad, sometimes you get used to the person. When you get into the routine and your mate is an addict, abusive or worse, you may leave them. But, even when separating you go forward then back and get stagnant. You just get familiar, the same thing, and the negatives of it. When you're used to it, it's hard to get out even when you have remorse. You choose to be happy about those little portions of goodness, you squeeze for dear life on the good things, even though they are far and few between, but it's not worth it...

Where it Starts

As a man, you know off the top when you make eye contact where it would go with that individual and yourself – to a conversation, to lunch, to dinner, or to the bedroom...

When a man sees a future he takes his time. You open the door for her and she unlocks the door for you...courting and dating...

People should take their time. Babies shouldn't have babies, they can't teach them things. They can't raise them or train them up in the way they should go. They can take care of them but they can't really teach them.

Blessed are the footsteps, which are ordered by God.

Losing "It"

"Give It to Me Baby" Rick James
"I Don't Love You Anymore" Teddy Pendergrass
"My Love (You're Never Gonna Get It)" En Vogue
"Just When We Start Making It" Tower of Power
"Bump & Grind" R. Kelly

"We forgot about tomorrow as we lay, didn't think about the price we had to pay." ~ Lyrics from "As We Lay," Shirley Murdock

So now you're in the relationship and things have been going reasonably well, right? And then the eyes start to wander, perhaps the texting and the computing starts to increase... and before you know it – sucked into "the drift" – you are sharing your relationship/mate with at least one other person – virtually or in reality.

We speak of virtually because it's easy and convenient to use social media and dating sites to get involved, infatuated, and caught up. It allows exes to look you up or strangers looking for love and you happen to be their target. "Innocently" igniting a spark and it begins a wicked cycle that becomes difficult to control, let alone, cut off.

Why does this happen? Ultimately, someone does not feel satisfied and they act out or act up, in this case. Ever heard of the song "I Can't Get No Satisfaction?" well sadly, it's true for many people. If you don't have a strong sense of self, you are not committed to your mate and to the relationship, and you aren't willing to do the work to maintain a good relationship, it will be impossible to "feel good" and to "want it" let alone, want to stay in it.

Resisting Temptation takes willpower, discipline, the sincere desire to keep your relationship, hard work, and also the ability and willingness to say no.

"If your mind and spirit is focused on your mate by them constantly making deposits – when I say deposits, insuring that you are constantly reminded of how plentiful, complete and equally yoked the relationship is it'll be easier to resist temptation.

However if your mate is not giving you what you need, it can cause problems. Physically being there, being able to add to the financial responsibilities, being able to help out with work situations, being accessible, even on the phone, able to give immediate responses, on the spot. Those are things that are important and necessary for me so having distance can also make it challenging." ~ Ice

"I disagree. I feel it's up to the person to be satisfied – and not put it on their mate. Both partners need and deserve deposits and if both partners have a solid foundation as individuals, they will realize the value of what they have; and take responsibility for their own role." ~ Water

"Why would you risk losing the relationship if your relationship is complete? You probably won't risk it if you have your needs met. There are guys out there who do have their needs met, they have everything they want and they still stray. If they do that, stay on the hunt, it's because they are having a hard time dealing with their own satisfaction, thus earning the label of 'dog'." ~ Ice

"That's a good question. Why would they? Too many people think it's better 'on the other side'" and they find out later that what they had was a blessing. If you're trying to do it all yourself, it's hard to resist what isn't good for you. That's where getting out of the flesh is important." ~ Water

STRATEGIC PLANNING FOR LOVE & WAR

What Can You Do About "The Drift?"

First, recognize when it's happening to you. Be honest with yourself and your mate. It could be about the beer belly, the hair curlers and flannel pajamas, the late nights at work, bad attitudes, boredom, stress, life, or even kids.

Ask if it's happening to your mate if you are sensing that she or he may be drifting, be an adult and ask a difficult question. "Baby, are you losing your desire for me?" "Am I still pleasing you?" "What could I do differently?" You may be afraid of the answers or the truth, but if you don't ask your mate, who can you ask? And if you don't ask your mate, you may be leaving a crack in the window or door for you or for them.

Be Real and Realistic

As we've said before, the source of conflict is often failed expectations. Think about it; if you know something in advance, you can often think about it and come to terms with it. However, when you "expect something" and it doesn't happen the way you think it should, those disappointments can become poisonous and cause disconnection.

Once the exuberance of the relationship has come down to earthly levels, it's almost as if the "shine" has worn off and you real-eyes your mate is not even close to being "perfect." They'll likely have some flaws, secrets, challenges, problems, and habits that you won't like.

Actually, you will too. Each of us has trucks full of issues that we bring with us and recognizing that, accepting that, and being willing to step up to working through them is key to halting the drift.

STRATEGIC QUESTIONS TO ASK YOURSELF WHEN CONSIDERING STAYING IN OR LETTING GO:

1. Do I like them?

2. Do I like the person I have become now that I'm with them?

3. Do I love them, for real? (For who he or she is and is not)

4. Do I see myself waking up to this person every single day for the next 30 years (especially in sickness and through major losses)?

5. Do I like the way I feel when I'm with them?

6. Do we bring out the best in each other or are we clinging to fear and not wanting to be "out there" alone?

7. What "failed" expectations might I need to let go of and forgive (regarding me, my mate, our relationship)?

8. How does our relationship affect others in our lives?

9. What do I expect once I'm single, if we break up?

10. Am I willing to change my own approach and work through things or have I passed the point of no return?

Self-Assessment

Once you've asked these questions, then do a self-assessment. There is something that is occurring to create the rift between you as a once harmonious couple. So, ask yourself what you may or may not being doing to contribute to the drift that is happening.

If I choose to stay, am I willing to check my ego and get in touch with, and accept the realities of where we both are today?

Everyone has limitations, imperfections, and limitless possibilities. Often our biggest struggles are internal. Stuff hurts then we naturally implore coping mechanisms to help ease the pain but those are usually temporary aides. Some people run to sex and some people run to the Bible. It's the way we've learned to relieve the pressure. Others turn to shopping, depression, gambling, lying, faking, drugs, avoidance, alcohol, or even abuse.

"'After you've done all you can, just stand,' as Donnie Mc Clurkin, sings. The reality is that as teens we probably thought we could conquer the world and that our best days were ahead of us. As we age, something shifts, if we let negativity and perceptions trick us into thinking 'it's too late to change' or 'I'm just tired.'" ~ Water

"Sure, you or your partner may not be as viral, 'hot' or driven as you once were however, once you become honest about your struggles with yourself first, and then with your mate, you will find that the shame, guilt, or pain are only covering the joy that is the real, true you." ~ Ice

Acknowledging who you are today is the first step to claiming your greatness. Being vulnerable allows the closing of some doors and also the opening of others. Be willing to work through things and you'll be amazed at what you may uncover.

Make some choices. Depending on where you are in life, make sure that you and your partner are going in the same direction and want similar things. Try new things. Communicate more, be trustworthy, flexible, and discuss what's not working so that you both can choose what you need to do – together to make it work.

In the lyrics of Mariah Carey, *"We Belong Together."*

New Booty, Cheating, and Perceptions

"Do Me Baby" Prince
"Pop That Thang" Isley Brothers
"Scandalous" Prince
"Nasty Girl" Vanity Six
"Whip Appeal" Babyface
"Ain't No Sunshine When She's Gone" Al Green

"There's nothing better than booty unless it's new booty…" Well, that's what "they say." And will they be there to pick up your broken pieces if you make a hasty dumb move? Stop in the name of love and think of the time that old booty was new to you.

"Tonight I Celebrate My Love" Peabo Bryson & Roberta Flack

You remember how your relationship was fresh and new? You were like Sonny & Cher singing, "*I Got You Babe.*" When the phone rang and you couldn't wait to talk to them? Or, you told them, "*I Just Called to Say I Love You,*" like Stevie Wonder. When you were just waiting for that date so you could get with them? Yeah, you used to be new. The smells, the way the hips moved? The passion the kisses ignited and the enthusiasm that charged through your body and soul that came with the newness? You were hopelessly devoted like Olivia Newton John! The excitement, goose bumps and thrills? The sexy undergarments? The times when your mate, and especially pleasing your mate was *the* priority?

Is it realistic to assume that the relationship can "stay new?" No. So, as long it is not your partner's expectation (because if they do expect new, you are in trouble anyway), do some

93

STRATEGIC PLANNING FOR LOVE & WAR

things to spice up your relationship for real. Things that you both can agree to and engage in, and make sure it's not just about the physical – because spiritual, emotional, and mental stimulation are all keys to having a successful relationship.

"Men do not govern their thoughts and movements through conversation. We aren't as thoughtful, compassionate or verbal with our communication as women are. And we don't make decisions based on our emotions.

Emotions play a big role for women, especially in relationships. That is why I feel there are women dating women relationships; they have those pieces. But even in those relationships you still find yourself dealing with insecurity, whether or not you will become the old versus the new, the young, the better shaped, you know the drill." ~ Ice

Why Do Men Cheat?

1. Because they can. That's one real answer. Now, let's get to some other possibilities.

2. Not satisfied anymore – perhaps he hasn't clearly communicated his desires to his mate. Or maybe he has clearly communicated and his spouse is not willing to do those things.

3. The woman changes – she used to be glamorous and dressed in nice open toed shoes and sun dresses or perhaps she got saved and changed her dress to go with her newfound religious walk.

4. The man feels the need to be desired and thinks he can find that in the bosom of another – perhaps he's going through a midlife crisis and needs to know that women still want him.

Sometimes people start cheating because they don't feel supported. Sometimes there's a rough patch and they don't feel harmony. Peace in the home is important.

We usually go somewhere when something is missing and then we can easily tell the other person exactly what our mate is not doing *right now* and so guess what? That's what the next person is going to do...

Don't run out to find someone to help you feel better – the other person can make you feel better to lure you in when you are vulnerable. It probably won't be worth it.

Fried chicken, peach cobbler and greens, designer purses, jewels, and perfume – the other person is going to have a game plan and 'get you' and then slowly, things are separating.

Have you been considering trading in your "old" model? Tune in to your real feelings. Don't "*Rock the Boat*" prematurely because "*Gigolos Get Lonely Too*."

Jodeci said it really well in their song "*Stay*" and begged for her to come back home. If you think, "new radio" is better than "old radio," keep in mind that the old one knows your music – your favorite station and songs. It is always faithful, it provides comfort, support, stability, and most of all, that feeling of appreciation, hitting just the right notes when you pay attention and listen.

Do yourself a favor and play "*Closer than Close*," by Atlantic Starr and let it remind you of the times when you felt like your love would last until the Universe would pass because the Whispers say, "*It's a Love Thing*."

We're Just Not There (Yet)?

"What You Won't Do for Love" Bobby Caldwell
"When We Get Married" Larry Graham
"Be My Girl" The Dramatics
"Love Don't Love Nobody" Spinners
"I Can't Help It" Michael Jackson
"Joy and Pain" Maze featuring Frankie Beverly

"I'm not a doctor or PhD, I'm here to offer real life perspective from a man's point of view, my own experiences, and most of all my heart. I want people to know that there's more to relationships than just giving compliments, paying bills, and being a father. Creating and maintaining successful relationships involves communication, giving, being considerate, and making personal sacrifices to make the relationship work." ~ Ice

"My purpose is to help people know how much they matter and that they have choices...I didn't get to having effective 'adult conversations' by accident or by intention; I've just had many conflicts (I'm pretty direct) and have learned the hard way (still learning!) the art of tact and diplomacy...I don't want others to make my mistakes!!!" ~ Water

Ice feels that women aren't aware of the "stages" that men have and Water feels that men should communicate differently. Many men will say, "I'm not married" yet, they hold "their woman" to certain standards. Many women will take what the man says and believe that "We are committed," and not engage in behaviors contradictory to that. This section is for your consideration, communication, and for you to open up about your own/your partner's expectations. Because if you view the "stages" differently, or don't even know they exist in your mate's mind, then according to Ice, their activities can be "perceived" as cheating.

"We have had plenty of discussions and experiences on this subject and to be honest, I'm still a little foggy about Ice's perspective and I don't know that I agree. However, Ice does share things the way he sees it. So ladies, I'm sure we'll be able to have some good discussions about this in our own circles and with the men we know." ~ *Water*

Ice Shares:

Women, please understand that a man has needs and it's important for everyone to stay in their lane. If you want to date and keep your options open then be on that page.

A lot of women get into what I feel is a no difference in the dating and the marriage mentality; they expect the same level. You need to understand this: it's not the same. There are three main stages that lead to the lifelong commitment. If you understand that this is where most men are coming from, it will help you make choices for yourself when it comes to the person you are seeing.

Stage One (Dating)

When you are dating, you are casually and conveniently seeing one another, you are getting together, having fun and getting to know each other. You both may or may not see other people but you may or may not have discussed it with the other person yet.

Stage Two (Girlfriend)

At this point you've said to each other, "I don't want to see anyone else but you" and you are both okay with that. When you are "in a relationship" you are building and finding out if you have a future, you are figuring out if you are compatible.

Things like, Are you neat like me? What's your family like? Do you pay your bills like me? Those are things you experience with your mate.

Some people think they know pretty quickly and get engaged or married after three to six months. Then six months to a year later that didn't work. You do hear of stories when it works, but most of the time it doesn't so, I'm skeptical.

You don't rush stuff, ladies especially; take your time when in this stage. Honestly, most men won't tell you this however:

"Expect the best but prepare for the worst. You should prepare for things not being what you think they may be."

This is happening because as you go through this stage, mini-tests are happening throughout the relationship. This helps a man figure out whether or not you are marriage material. The trust and the level of the relationship may not be what you thought it was; or you may think you want something to be different and either or both of you may not be living up to certain expectations.

At this point the status may change and someone may pull back. That's usually where the breakdown happens. The partner may or may not communicate with you and may feel like they want to see someone else because it's not all that they want but they may not tell you this.

"This is where I have the issue — you discussed the agreement with the other person and now he wants to pull back, but you are all caught up. You need to be able to pull back too, hang in there or walk away because he can't make up his mind about what he is going to do with you." ~ Water

"*He knows; a man has his own process. He may just not have reached the point where you may be. But he knows. He has already determined after the mini-tests if he can see you as his wife. So until he is ready to propose or move to that level, he's comfortable. If he can't see you as his wife, he may ride it out; or until you get fed up; or until he just doesn't want to be in the relationship.*

He may not communicate and speak about it so you need not to pay attention to what he's saying — base it on what he's doing." ~ Ice

"*This is the danger zone. This is exactly what I'm saying about being unclear. If we are in a relationship and we're seeing each other exclusively and now he's pulling back, how is a woman to know if he's pulling out or if he's slowing down to prepare?*

Especially if he's now 'keeping options open' and changing the agreement (i.e. seeing other people)? As a woman, you have to make a decision if it's worth waiting, adjusting or letting go of the relationship if that happens." ~ Water

Stage Three (My Woman/Wife)

When it's time for marriage, if it's time for marriage, it will happen. You don't have to force it and you don't have to run shotgun on anyone. Some people don't have the defense mechanism to stop it or to speak up for themselves.

Both parties, and namely the man, feels like the situation is right and that "This time, I'm all in and I'm going to be with this one for the rest of my life because I know that this is the right thing. I respect her, I love her and I want to be with her."

"*Why are men usually the one(s) to propose?*" ~ Water

"*Dealing with tradition. There's nothing anywhere that says that a woman can't propose to a guy. Women are more likely to be ready*

99

to settle down and have the level of commitment. Most men struggle with that and it will take a little while to come around, I admit that. Because they don't have everything out of their system yet. Why would I put myself in that level of commitment if I'm not ready for that?" ~ Ice

"Yet, men will often represent that they are ready to be in that relationship and as women feel 'secure' that you are working toward marriage. This is where it's easy to get caught up and hurt.

What should women do to protect themselves or to make sure that they don't have false expectations?" ~ Water

"Take it slow. And even though things seem okay on the surface, don't just go with that. 'Oh, he takes care of his kids.' 'Oh, he has good credit and a good job.' That's not enough. Make sure you find out 'What kind of individual is he?' 'What relationship does he have with his family?' 'What about his character?' Get to know him. Just because he seems to meet your qualifications, you must still give it time. See how you handle adverse times together. Notice how he treats you, things like that.

Women need to slow down. I'm not saying take five to 10 years, that's not fair. It's worth insuring that you have the best candidate, and even more importantly, the best 'willing' candidate." ~ Ice

"Interesting." ~ Water

Patience or Pressure

"If you are looking for a companion, fun, mutual respect, to be spiritually connected, it's worth waiting for...If you force it or speed it up, you'll get with someone out of season." ~ Ice

Pheromones

"After the Dance" Marvin Gaye
"Special Lady" Ray, Goodman & Brown
"Love You Down" Ready for the World
"Shake Your Pants" Cameo
"Caught My Eye" Mint Condition
"Back in Love (Everytime I Turn Around)" LTD

pher•o•mone noun \ ˈfer-ə-ˌmōn\

: a chemical substance that is usually produced by an animal and serves especially as a stimulus to other individuals of the same species for one or more behavioral responses

Definition from Merriam-Webster.com/dictionary

A man shares his thoughts about attraction, passion and the acting out on those instincts, from his point of view.

When a man is attracted to a woman, even though she may be a perfect stranger, the psychological reaction is powerful, overwhelming, and almost irresistible.

When the pheromones are working, he shows her that he is gentle and strong. He will not hurt you, but he does exert and the balance is beautiful. That is where he shares his love.

If a man is in a relationship and he gets together with another woman, it doesn't mean he doesn't necessarily love the woman he's with. There exists an animalistic nature, which is meant to create. There is a sort of primitive act of dominance that a man feels when it is triggered by the pheromones. He's attracted to the eyes, to the touch, to the scent and if the scent is good to you, you have to conquer it.

It is not this worldly — it's peeling off the panties, feeling you, and the act of submission. It doesn't mean he doesn't love the person

that he loves; I'm not saying it's right — the visual takes over; then she smiles and she shows she's open; it's the first, second, and then third look if you are compatible; then it's the scent of the breath, it's the pheromones; then by the time you finally get to the sense of your femininity then that's it...we try to make it intellectual.

Monogamy takes maturity. Wealth means you can do what you want. The poor are so poor they don't care. For women there is some maturity, as they grow older. There is so much responsibility for a man — once he accepts it however, then he becomes the patriarch.

Often when people get divorced, someone is growing and someone is not growing; then there's no communication; then no sex; then it opens the door for someone else to come into the picture because they look right, they smell right, and then it's too late.

Couples must stay engaged. If both sides are actually taking care of each other, because we are paying attention and embracing the newness and we aren't jealous of the newness and we still want to chase each other around the room and enjoy one another, we have something. We are willing to try new things whatever it is, changing the way you dress or the way you wear your hair.

Change your approach and appreciate what he does; don't nag and simply love him and acknowledge him for what he does. This is a good antidote — that's so much better. Changing your attitude and being real, while you are appreciating him, will inspire him to do the things you'd like him to do. Ask him "What do you think?" by asking his input he will also feel appreciated because he gets a chance to please his woman.

He knows she needs something from him, and he feels needed and it's more than just the sex...don't be fake because he will recognize that.

Men won't tell you this but they want a woman who makes him feel like he needs to earn it. ~ Mr. D.J.

DANGER

WATCH YOURSELF AND YOUR BACK.

Thrills are often short lived but can have serious consequences.

Stalkers!

"Back Stabbers" The O'Jays
"Baby I'm Scared of You" Womack & Womack
"Get the Funk out My Face" Brothers Johnson
"Dangerous" Michael Jackson
"Poison" Bell, Biv, DeVoe
"Crazy in Love" Beyonce

She could be around the corner, she could be down the street, but most of all beware that she *could be* where you sleep.

"I was watching a 'Reality TV' show and the husband put a GPS tracker on his wife's cell phone because he thought she was cheating. I did not know those (phone devices) even existed. He showed up where she was rehearsing. She didn't know how he knew where she was because she didn't tell him. One day at home she was telling him how her phone had been acting funny and he came clean about what he did and of course, he had no remorse... A little back story, he cheated on her for five years of their eight-year marriage and he thinks that she is paying him back by cheating on him. People will go to all kinds of extremes. She got a new phone."
~ Mrs. Thomas

When you are in the relationship certain things may happen that can seemingly be explained away. However, you need to be clear about the *Warning Signs*. If you notice any of these things happening while you are in the relationship, she (or he, for that matter) may be a stalker disguised as the "love" of your life.

STRATEGIC OBSERVATIONS FOR NOTICING STALKER TENDENCIES

1. One day, after a minor disagreement your car is scratched.

2. You look through your drawers and some photos and other little knick-knacks seem to be missing and you think, maybe they are just misplaced. (They may already be destroyed or in that pile of the stalkers area waiting to be used in the future.)

3. You have conversations and your partner seems to know things that you don't remember discussing with them.

4. You notice that your female mate is taking "vitamins" and says they are to enhance certain body parts; or somehow the condoms keep coming up with holes in them.

5. Your friends stop inviting you to hang out or come to couple events because they don't feel comfortable with your mate – or they just don't like her or him.

"Be careful, pay attention to their behavior, and take your time. Get to know your mate. Don't jump into a situation just because it seems greener on the other side. Allow the relationship to mature. Be sure that the person lives up to their words and that their actions are consistent." ~ Ice

Permanent relationships deserve as much certainty as possible.

Blood and War

"Bad Habits" Maxwell
"Stranger" LTD
"Crazy" Rahsaan Patterson
"Billie Jean" Michael Jackson
"Better Days" Dianne Reeves
"Humpin'" The Gap Band
"Sadie" The Spinners

Bad habits and bad behaviors often run in families. *They say* that the way a man treats his mother is the way he'll treat his woman. That may or may not be true.

Men and Mothers

What about the way his mother treated him while he was growing up? What if she punched him, exposed him to her exploits with a new "uncle" every month, cussed incessantly, and dogged out his daddy every chance she got, or got hooked on drugs? Or, how about if she stayed in an abusive marriage or partnership throughout his life and he grew up hating the man who beat his mother and hating his mother for letting that man do it to her?

If the mother was an abuser or chronically addicted to substance, food, negativity or bad habits, maybe he's just hurt, disgusted or frankly scared as hell to trust another woman? Maybe he hasn't learned how to function in a healthy, loving way with women. Isn't that possible?

Mama's Boys

"Mama's boy, that's a cop out." ~ Ice

106

Ladies, when you come across that situation, you need to approach it in a way that you are letting mom know that you have his best interests in mind. Communicate "I am not here to take him away from you, I'm here for us as a family to evolve, get better and get stronger," in words, body language, and in attitude.

You want to relax her motherly posture. You want her to scale back, not have the reigns on him become tighter; you want them to become looser. Mom needs to know that she is respected and that her son has a real woman in his life. Otherwise you will always be at war with the mother.

"Some men need to grow the hell up. I understand that's your mom but you have to stand up on your own two feet and her job is done. The things she has shown you, now it's time to show her that you are putting to use the nurturing, love, and respect. This is my girlfriend, my woman, my wife (as you get through those levels of your relationship) and I need you to respect that." ~ Ice

Apples and Trees

They also say that the apple doesn't fall far from the tree. That may or may not be true. How did this person grow up and where are they going? *"I Wanna Sex You Up"* is what you may be thinking when you see that big butt and a smile. *"I Want Muscles"* when you see those arms and abs. But don't complain when your *"Love Jones"* creates an 18-year contract with someone who has a bad attitude, no job, and no real future for themselves, let alone for your little rugrats.

Jack and Jill went up the hill and now they have a son and a daughter. Then you're stuck – welcome to your inheritance!

Interview your mate and get to the heart of the matter and the truth. You both deserve to know about family histories because issues like mental illness, past trauma, as well as physical, emotional, and substance abuse will affect your relationship – directly or indirectly.

Vapors of a Vibrant Woman

Mother figures, biological or not, are some of the biggest influences on entire families, let alone children. Men play a huge role in the 'health' of women as well because based on the way a relationship goes, the woman may or may not 'bounce back' or remain vibrant especially after relationships filled with conflict, strife, or constant battles. Though full of love for her grandmother, who brought her up, one woman shares:

"I felt like I was going to lose my mind one day and just snap. I was afraid that I would end up shriveled, mean, lonely, and bitter just like her..." My big mama raised me and she just stayed in the house all day, the doctors had said she was depressed.

I remember how pretty she was, full of life, talent, and the will to live. She was fun and used to sing songs, dance, and teach us stuff. I think it was that last relationship with the 'unavailable guy' that finally took her over the edge.

'Where did she go?' She was full of medicine, pain, anger, and unresolved hurt. I thank God for that little cat of hers because I think Peachy was the only thing that would get her out of bed most days. Well actually, Peachy and running out of cigarettes. Storms, disasters, the sun, people who loved her, birthdays, running out of food or medicine, none of those really moved her to leave the house; until she was close to her last puff and then in the car she went.

It hurt me to be around her because it's like I couldn't help her — she was just stuck and I felt helpless to do anything for her 'cause she didn't even act like she wanted to help herself.' Then one day I looked in the mirror and said to myself, 'She scares me because I'm afraid I'll become her.' " ~ Marie

The Future

The likelihood of becoming a caregiver to your mate, your parents, or your in-laws (legal or not) is a reality in today's world. It's a good idea to get to know what comes along with your package. We are not encouraging you to run away. Sometimes you are the very answer that the love of your life needs. Maybe you are the friend, and your unconditional love is an answer to prayer. Perhaps being with you after years of heartache is the reward for holding on to life. If being with you represents the first time that person can truly love and be loved in return, then understand how delicate that balance is — along with the honor and responsibility that comes with sharing the best of who you are.

STRATEGIC REFLECTION FAMILY RELATIONSHIP QUESTIONS

1. How do they respond to dramatic experiences?
2. Do they shut down and stop speaking?
3. Do they fly off the handle and start hitting?
4. Do they start to withhold sex?
5. Do they stop their normal behavior?
6. Do they transform into a Cyber Stalker by jumping into your email and social media accounts?

7. Do they "punish you" as if you were a child or behave in verbally or physically aggressive ways?

8. Did they have traumatic experiences while growing up that may be affecting them now? If so, are they willing to get help/counseling?

9. Are you prepared to love your mate through/in spite of the past?

In your 20's or 30's actions and expectations should be different than in your 40's or 50's. Where you are in life will probably affect your tolerance and maturity level.

"We Are Family" Sister Sledge

Down Low

"Trapped in the Closet" R. Kelly
"Keep It on the Down Low" R. Kelly featuring Ron Isley
"He Brought Me Out" Billy Preston
"If I Were a Boy" Beyonce
"The Rain" Oran "Juice" Jones
"Creepin'" Luther Vandross

When certain men identify themselves as heterosexual, but have sex with men; and then avoid sharing this information even if they have female sexual partner(s) it's dangerous, unfair, and not okay.

"Trapped in the Closet" along with the accompanying video series, is an example of how when one person sneaks around, others are exposed – literally. By the time you follow the string of seemingly unending twists, turns, lies, sex partners, cheaters and such, news of the "package" is devastating to the wife of the minister who became dis-eased. The hurt, pain, and the consequences of this risky behavior is frightening.

"Down Low is the ultimate deception. If you know you are a man and you want to be a provider, a leader with your woman, or you know you are gay and you know that's what you want, then be that.

Men, imagine being a woman and you are the head of the household, an alpha male. She respects you, caters to you, and gives you everything you need to feel that you matter. And lo and behold she comes home one day and you are in the bedroom getting down with another man.

I hope by reading this scenario it helps you to think about your actions. If you can really put yourself in her shoes, how would you feel? So just call it what it is; you are gay or you are straight, just be a man. Don't hide and run your household based on a lie." ~ Ice

Be honest and don't hurt people because you are too cowardly to admit your sexual preference. If you or your lover is knowingly engaged in this type of behavior, grow up, come clean, and make "responsible" choices.

Don't Be Lazy!

"Gotta Go, Gotta Leave" Vivian Green
"Tired of Being Alone" Al Green
"Tears" Force MDs
"The Blues" Tony Toni Tone

Ants are a great example of wisdom, hard work, and ingenuity. They know what they need and provide it. In the summer they have plenty. In the fall they have a harvest. Ants are constantly and consistently working for and toward their best interest.

For humans, it's okay to sleep. A little rest is good, especially following periods of focused work. Yet, do not allow yourself to slumber into laziness; it ends in poverty and becoming complacent. Lazy will come if you don't have a mind to be good and do good.

Lazy in Relationships

Don't forget what got you here today. You met as two individuals and you became one. The person you were, that attracted your mate to you, needs to continue to be in the relationship or it won't last.

For example, if you used to bring flowers, cook four times a week, had sex three times a week, went to church weekly while you were dating, helped kids with homework, spent quality time, you need to keep those things up because otherwise your relationship will slowly end.

"Stay mindful, never lazy, always be a willing participant. Stay self-motivated, highly effective, and promote positive reinforcements." ~ Ice

"Don't be so self-centered that you are not mindful of your partner's needs, desires, and wants. It's easy to be on your own plan so much that you leave the other person out in the cold." ~ Water

Changes

Beyond mental laziness, changes can happen. If you can't do some of those things you used to because physically things have changed...then get help.

If one of the partners is having trouble in the sex department, there may be reasons – medical reasons. So, if the man says he doesn't want to, it may be because the blood isn't circulating like it used to and he doesn't want to tell you. Go to the doctor and get checked out. It could be the onset of diabetes or high blood pressure. Or perhaps for women it was having a child and losing the desire.

Jobs change, funds change, and so if circumstances change, that's different. If you "bought your relationship" you are in trouble. If you were to become disabled and your relationship was based on material and the physical, you will be in trouble. Keep it in mind.

Timing can affect things too so make sure everything is okay with both of you. Consider counseling if trying to do it on your own isn't working; please don't be stubborn and get it all checked out. Your relationship is worth it, right?

When people become lazy they talk "slickly" and "take shortcuts." Things that used to be standard expectations are lost. People don't take responsibility for their actions or for the actions of others. These short cuts have short-circuited skills, minds, families, and behavior! Being good and doing good!

Pre-Commitment Check List

"Shining Star" Earth, Wind & Fire
"Somethin' Special" The Temptations
"The Knowledge" Janet Jackson
"Sweet Thing" Chaka Khan
"Thriller" Michael Jackson
"The Answer Is You" Phyllis Hyman
"Then Came You" Dionne Warwick and the Spinners

If you really want a relationship worth having, and to avoid a catastrophic war later on, you must be willing to ask and give honest answers to issues that will affect each partner in the long run.

Since choosing your life partner is one of the most important decisions you'll ever make, here are some questions for your checklist.

Even if you are currently in the relationship, this list is important to consider because perhaps you don't know the honest answers to these questions, and others like them. Take the time to fill in the gaps. After all, your relationship is worth having, right?

STRATEGIC PLANNING QUESTIONS PRIOR TO MAKING COMMITMENTS

1. Are you in a current relationship? (And, what's the real status?)

2. Do you have children? Do you want children? How do you feel about children? (Do you like them? Do you like to be around them? Etc.)

3. How's your credit score? Are there liens or settlements against you?

4. Are there any current, past convictions, or warrants against you?

5. Are you or have you been a drug user? (Prescription or otherwise?)

6. How often do you drink adult beverages?

7. What are your feelings about celibacy and "safe" sex?

8. How often do you like to have sex?

9. Do you have any STDs?

10. What is your HIV status?

11. Do you have any other potentially long-term health challenges?

12. What's your overall physical (and mental) health? Do you get regular mammograms, prostate checks, pap smears, blood work, regular physicals, etc.?

STRATEGIC PLANNING QUESTIONS REGARDING CHILDREN

1. Do you have children?

2. How do you feel about introducing children (yours or mine) in new dating situations?

3. How is your relationship with your ex? (Is it harmonious, non-existent, communicative, "complicated" or are you at war?)

4. How might that communication affect our relationship?

5. What are your concerns about children (yours or mine), as they relate to us as a couple?

If these questions are too much for you to bear, then maybe you are not ready to be in a real relationship with them or maybe they aren't right for you.

Blinded by Love… Grown and Not Mature

"You're a Big Girl Now" Stylistics
"Is It Still Good To Ya?" Ashford & Simpson
"You're Still a Young Man" Tower of Power
"I Just Want It to Be Over" Keyshia Cole
"Grown & Sexy" Babyface
"Ooh Child" Five Stairsteps

Sometimes after a female gives birth, she thinks she can handle all that life offers and thinks she doesn't have to be accountable to anyone. Well, especially when she has children, she has a duty and obligation to make good choices and to *not* allow a man to bring her down. Here's a situation that one young woman is facing…if only this was an isolated incident…

What are two of the biggest problems that people face in relationships?

I think the biggest problems are trust and money issues.

Do you think it's based on the person being insecure, selfish, or just not caring about the other person?

I think it is being selfish, and not caring. My stepdaughter's boyfriend does it to her all the time but she is blinded by love. He doesn't work. He stays at home all day playing video games and watching the kids sometimes. Before she met him she had two jobs and a car. Now she has a job working at a second hand store, with no car because he won't let her work where he can't walk in and see her.

Wow. How old are they? Why do you think she is allowing him to treat her that way?

She is 23 and he is 24. She just got her income tax check back on Monday (6 days ago), and it was a large sum. Friday the water and the lights got cut off. Today is Sunday and he has already spent half of it.

I don't understand why that is happening. How old are the children? Where is her father in this (your husband)? What are you doing to help her? Does anyone talk to her / tried to get her to leave him?

We have all tried to talk to her, but she says she's grown and can handle it. She has two kids, a 1-year-old and a 3-year-old. His parents don't want to have anything to do with him because he steals and lies and that is how he keeps conning her. She gets food stamps and he sells them and she won't say anything to him about it, then she comes to us, and wants to borrow money to get food, and diapers. Otherwise, she will go over to her grandmother's and eats what food she wants and then take it home but the grandmother told her the other day that this has to stop.

She was living in an apartment, paying no rent and he decided he wanted to sell liquor out of the apartment and got caught. Then they had to move. At this moment, the four of them are staying in a one bedroom apartment. They found out yesterday that they have to move because she lied on the application and said it was for her and one kid. The leasing office found out that he and the other child were living there and that he was selling drugs, so they have to move next week.

Her father is here, but you know kids when they think they are grown. We have tried to help her, but as long as we help her, he won't do anything because he knows we are going to help her and the kids. So he refuses to work and she lets him stay there and not do anything.

Source: Facebook Interview with PJ

Comments:

Experience and time will reveal because for whatever reason she is blinded by the "love," the looks, or perhaps the sex. If a man is not being a father or the leader, you must choose to lose him.

STRATEGIC PLANNING PRODUCTIVITY QUESTIONS

Especially For Women

1. Why am I still with him?
2. What is he doing to support our family?
3. How do I feel about myself, our kids and about him?
4. How are my actions endangering the welfare of (our) children?
5. How are my actions affecting the other people in our lives?

Especially For Men

1. Do I respect myself?
2. Am I living up to my own goals and dreams?
3. How do I feel about myself when I look in the mirror?
4. What has happened to me that makes me okay with living this way?
5. What steps am I willing to take to be positive, productive and mature?

Ask these questions first of yourself. Be honest. Then ask your partner to answer. Be open to listening to his/her honesty. Think back to what you used to do. Are you still making the same choices, and the same mistakes? If the answer is yes, it's time to stop.

4 am Beat Down

"Seven Whole Days" Toni Braxton
"Killing Me Softly with His Song" Roberta Flack
"Killing Me Softly with His Song" The Fugees
"I'm Going Down" Rose Royce
"I'm Going Down" Mary J. Blige
"I Will Survive" Gloria Gaynor
"Blame It" Jamie Foxx

"Tony then grabbed me by the neck, turned me around, and slammed me against my car. He punched me several times in my face and when I dropped to the ground he kicked me over and over again. I knew this was it for me. It was almost 4 in the morning, no one was out at this time, and my phone had been thrown in a sewer; I couldn't even make an emergency call. I didn't need a mirror to see that, once again, my face was a mess. Tony threw my car keys on the ground and he walked away, leaving me there. I felt the warm blood from my nose run from my face and watched as it drained in the same sewer my phone had been thrown. I was able to pick myself up once again and drive home.

I was a victim of what most would describe as domestic abuse. I was too embarrassed to say anything to anyone and therefore have kept it a secret until now. Falling on the ground was much easier than rising up again." ~ *Aigner Martin, excerpt from her book "Perseverance is Remembrance."*

Too many people find themselves in living nightmares. It starts with a look, a nod, or a stare. It escalates to a few chosen words and then before you know it, "Pow! Bam! Kick." Certainly there are people who chronically abuse others and if you are seeing, feeling, or noticing behaviors don't take them lightly. This is true for you and for friends and family members alike. Too many times people feel isolated, ashamed alone and are silent, perhaps even suicidal.

Becoming a victim is never intentional but staying a victim can become addictive. And then it becomes a pattern, just like the abuser.

There are many types of abuse and it can occur in different ways. When we hear about abuse we often think about physical abuse and stalking, but there are so many different types and it's all serious. No one deserves to be abused. Other types include Emotional/Verbal Abuse, Financial Abuse, Sexual Abuse, and Digital Abuse (using texting and social networking to monitor, bully or intimidate a partner through technology.)

People often stay in these relationships because of conflicting emotions like fear, believing abuse is normal, embarrassment, low self-esteem, love, and pressure (from peers, elders, or for cultural or religious reasons).

Too many times people won't leave because they feel a reliance on the abusive partner. If you think you won't have enough money or nowhere to go, it leads to deeper feelings of isolation and helplessness.

If you are being abused, get help. And, if you think someone you know is being abused, reach out and offer support, love, tangible help, and no judgment.

The National Domestic Violence Hotline is 1-800-799-7233 or www.TheHotline.Org is a great source of information for anyone who has considerations, questions, or needs. All calls to the National Domestic Violence Hotline are anonymous and confidential.

Take this time to reflect. Understand that the physical, mental, verbal, sexual abuse is not by any means a substitute or an excuse for love. This is a simply act of control. Not so much of the relationship but of you, this type of person wants to have absolute power over you.

"Get to understand the characteristics of this particular person, and please do not ignore the red flags. If they have 'put you isolation' from friends and family, that is a key element down the wrong road, and is a sign of abuse. You do have a choice and if you don't take the time to get to know someone, you can be in ill-treated, misunderstood, and have a distorted idea that it's about love but it's not. It's about control, rooted in their own fear.

Smoke screens wrapped in 'I didn't mean to break your jaw' or 'force you into...' Put an ill-placed cloud that has you thinking it's love but it's beyond love and war, it's about your life. Don't put or keep yourself in potentially life-threatening situations for anyone or anything." ~ Ice

A Woman's Position on Cheating from a Man's Perspective

"Chick on the Side" Pointer Sisters
"Irreplaceable" Beyonce
"It's a Thin Line Between Love and Hate" The Pretenders
"It's a Thin Line Between Love and Hate" H-Town
"Whenever You're Around" Jill Scott

PURPOSE – To help men understand where women are coming from when men cheat.

"The lack of sensitivity and the emotional boundaries that are involved are complicated and deep when a man cheats. When you are creating a safe haven for another that is considered cheating. Cheating is not just a physical act – it can also be what you think, what you do and time that you spend with another." ~ Ice

Time, communication, and attention are also considered cheating because these acts, even if they don't or haven't yet, crossed into physical/romantic gestures are like foreplay. They cross the boundaries of intimacy that she feels should be reserved exclusively for your relationship with her. She loses respect and trust for you and then lines of communication are broken. In the aftermath, it's the way she looks at you that can be forever altered because you are affecting so many things by your choices.

Healing & Forgiving: There are 4 stages that a woman goes through once she finds out that you have cheated.

1. **Disbelief** – *"I can't believe you stepped outside of our relationship situation."*

2. **Anger** – Sh*t hits the fan. *"The fact that you did it and the fact that I showed you that you didn't have to. You are a lowdown dirty MF not worthy of my respect or this family, you don't even respect yourself!"*

3. **Self-Assessment** – She's probably trying to re-enact what happened and analyze what is possibly missing. She's may now be trying to show him that she is capable of giving him what he thought he was missing.

4. **Relationship Worthy** – In her mind she is weighing the pros and cons of staying together. She's trying to figure out and thinking if it's worth forgiving him but not forgetting. She's considering to either stay with her man to grow and learn from the experience, or to constantly use that as a control measure and a constant reminder of how he disrespected the relationship.

The Choice

The flip side of using it as a control measure is to learn and to build a better relationship based on better communication, cohesiveness, and a change of behavior (no more cheating!).

Healing and Forgiving

You can't determine how long it's going to take for her to get over it because the stages are complicated – there's no time limit. So, if you step out, you have to be willing to weather the storm.

A Woman's Position on Her Man (Possibly) Cheating from a Woman's Heart

"It Hurts Like Hell" Aretha Franklin
"If Your Heart Isn't in It" Atlantic Star
"You Know That I Love You" Donell Jones
"End of the Road" Boyz II Men
"Giving You the Best that I've Got" Anita Baker
"Movin' Down the Line" Raphael Saadiq

"The thought of him cheating rocks my world. The thought of him calling, texting, or talking to another when I'm around or not makes me sick to my stomach. I can't change him, who he is, or what he does. I also know that I'm giving him the best that I've got. I know I'm not like other women from his past. I really thought he loved me and wants to be with me. I now realize I'm fragile. I thought I was bold and confident in our relationship, in our bond. I don't have the energy to threaten, cajole, try to control, or search for who and how these activities may be happening.

I know he has a good heart and a loving soul. I don't think that it's me, I don't know how to treat him better, this is the best I've ever done. If he's not satisfied, what can I really do about it? He's handsome, charming, warm, and engaging. What woman wouldn't want some of that? I just don't and can't share.

I hold my friends to standards — my man should be held to them as well. Now, we've made it around Facebook. I have incorporated him into my entire life and to think that my loving care is not enough. I don't have enough left for anger; I don't want to control; and I don't want to look over my shoulder everyday thinking is she 'the one?'" ~ Lady L.

Options and Choices

"Options...When your man says, 'I haven't seen her because I've been busy,' not because it's wrong, hurtful, or because I'm committed to you, it's more than a red flag, it's a bang on the head.

I asked him flat out, 'Oh, it's not because of me?' 'No,' he said. I said why are you talking to her and he said, 'Every since our status changed.' I said what do you mean? He said, 'Options.'

At that moment I thought 'Damn. What in the hell am I doing? And why is he in my damn bed? Get the heck out. I'm not going to be an option. It's not acceptable.' And then we went to sleep." ~ *Water*

STRATEGIC OBSERVATIONS AND CHEATING YELLOW FLAGS

1. He's been holding his phone so close to him, I have noticed it but, out of respect and to avoid problems or conflict, I have tried not to let it mean anything.

2. Thinking and admitting, "I'm afraid of what I may see." They say, that if you look for trouble, you will find it.

3. They also say, "Once a cheater, always a cheater." I don't want speculation and I do want the truth from him.

4. When you constantly think, "Why is this happening? I can't concentrate." And that feeling in the pit of your stomach doesn't go away.

STRATEGIC ALTERNATIVES TO COUNTERACTING CHEATING

1. Leave him and don't look back.

2. Cuss him out, cut up his clothes and put him out.

3. Act like you don't know and let things escalate.

4. Talk about him like a dog to your single friends and let them help you break up with him quicker.

5. Talk with him about it. If he really loves you and is committed to you and the relationship, he will likely tell you how he feels – and be prepared to hear his truth; it may or may not feel good at the time but may help you make the right decision for you.

6. Pray and wait for your answers.

"Say Amen" Howard Hewett

If you have done all you can do mentally, physically, emotionally, and spiritually, in the end, once you have given your best, you can walk away with your head held high. Don't let your relationship hold you captive, be willing to release, let go and remember, it's only (possibly) cheating.

When You Suspect Cheating

"It's the God in Me" Mary Mary
"Stand" Donnie McClurkin
"Come Back to Me" Janet Jackson
"I Want You Back" The Jackson Five
"I Heard it Through the Grapevine" Marvin Gaye

A Married Woman Shares...

"I knew some things and chose not to see...Unfaithfulness happened when we were dating and I didn't jump ship then. And honestly, even if I had put my foot down then, I don't know if it would be any different. I chose to stay in it. I have gone through stages of insecurity, low self-esteem and have questioned myself as a woman. And that question is, 'Why am I not good enough?'

I eventually left home because I got talked down to and then there was the verbal abuse and threat of physical abuse. It was too much. After I was gone for a while, he made changes within himself and his behavior. This changed the dynamic of our relationship and I went back home.

Things are a lot better. Of course, everyone is fallible but, our family is in tact and it's a lot better.

As a result of staying in it I'm more observant, I ask more questions and I pretty much don't stand for the b.s. anymore." Mrs. Barry

If you choose to remain involved in your relationship after you suspect that your partner may be cheating, you may need help – if you want to truly move forward.

If you really want to remain in your relationship, but you want real answers to help you make the healthiest decision for you, understand that may mean walking away at the end of the day.

"Jesus, You're the Center of My Joy" Richard Smallwood
"Order My Steps in Your Word" Mississippi Mass Choir

A woman used this journal entry/prayer to help remedy her suspicions and it worked for her. Be forewarned though, men and women, when you ask to be SHOWN, you may not like the realities of what you will see...

Prayer for Clarity

Lord, what's missing? If he's really my husband, I don't think he would put himself or me into compromising positions. I've also heard so many horror stories of women ignoring what they feel — choosing not to see.

What would you have me do and how would you have me do it?

I need You Lord. Please help me in the name of Jesus Christ. My whole future is wrapped up in this. Show me your way and help me to be obedient to your will, your desires for my life, destiny and future, and please bless him and us.

Please work to and through him and help him to be the man who you created him to be.

Lift him Father in his short-comings, in his prayer life, in his actions, thoughts, behaviors, dealings with others, and especially in his dealings with women, and with me. Please reveal to me what I should and need to know, all of it Lord.

God, please show me what I should do or not do. This is hard and I ask for strength and courage to make good choices and to please you.

I don't want to question him and I don't want to question my faith and right now I'm falling. Please help me Lord God, in Jesus name. I love and need you.

Your Child

HEALING

HEALING IS A PROCESS, NOT USUALLY A DESTINATION.

Pain, dis-ease and bad experiences can cloud your
life, your judgment, your outlook,
and your future.

Healing Matters

"Not Gon Cry" Mary J. Blige
"When You Love Someone" Maze featuring Frankie Beverly
"It Ain't No Use" Stevie Wonder
"Forever in Your Eyes" Mint Condition
"Kiss of Life" Sade

"I'm supposed to be evolving not revolving. So, a few years ago I changed my number and let the dead weight go." ~ Dionna J.

How to Live Through It

It's easy to repeat the same mistakes again and again – it's our patterns, our autopilot. At the end of the day, pain is what drives many people – to or from relationships and themselves.

Fear, horrific, terrifying fear can crumble the biggest economies, the most efficient systems and the seemingly solid relationships that we have.

If all you know is pain, doing things to figure out how to get past your pain, hurt and fear by dealing with the root cause of these things is important to building healthy relationships with others.

It Usually Takes Time and Help to Heal

If you never deal with issues from your past, the scabs become thick and cannot be penetrated. You will have roadblocks, more disappointments, and will struggle to get or maintain what you really want and deserve. So, when you acknowledge the pain, fear, anger or frustration, and admit that you want something better, that's an excellent first step.

"I was in a bad relationship and over the course of the 1 ½ years I gained 60 pounds. I didn't realize it at the time. But I was using food as my crutch versus alcohol, drugs, faith, or friendships to get me through. I found support when I met a personal trainer who helped me get healthy. Sure, we started with a meal plan and an exercise plan, but what really did it was the support, the caring, and the sense of belonging I felt. When I wanted to give up, she would call me and not take my excuses as an answer. It took less than four months to lose the weight because I wanted to be healed and was ready to do the work.

I also know that I need a plan for every day, for the rest of my life because my body, mind, and emotions are tied to my spirit." ~ *Vanessa P.*

You are not alone. Remember that, and don't isolate yourself even if you feel sad, unworthy, ashamed, or confused. Author Monikah Ogando-Halsey says, "Be soft on your past and hard on your future." Everyone "acts up" however; once you realize that you have been "acting up" by settling for less than you deserve, have stayed in a situation too long, or are still reeling from the past, remember that as long as you have breath, you have a new chance to start again.

Intimate Moments:
Desire and Wandering

"On the Ocean" K'Jon
"I Want You" Marvin Gaye
"Let's Get It On" Marvin Gaye
"Yearning for Your Love" Gap Band
"Intimate Friends" Eddie Kendricks

As Marvin Gaye's, "Distant Lover" plays in the background, my tears fall.

I promise Lord God that I try to stand tall.

Please help me to be humble and patient. You and only You know the true desires of my heart.

As I leave this place, my home of years, I pray, Oh Lord, that you fill my empty space.

It's been so long — yet has it ever been — that I have loved and been loved as you would have me be? Oh my Father, I just know that it's meant to be.

I am brave. I am strong. I will hold on. Please protect me and guide me as I start afresh — I wish to be strength and love and wisdom and faith.

My desire is to exercise my faculties — mind, body, and soul — and to fulfill all of your goals.

My vision has been limited and talents yet to be discovered. I wish to uncover that which you have given — and most of all I wish to give and be forgiven.

If only I could say — shoot, all I can do is pray this day — that You will continue to lead and guide and remind.

Perfect health — physically, mentally and spiritually. Love, peace and prosperity perpetually. Praise and joy continually.

Oh Lord Jehovah, I need You. Holy Spirit, I invite You. Jesus, in Your name, I Pray. No more waste. No more haste. Satisfaction. Peace of mind and peace of heart. Purpose. Wholeness. Completion. My husband. My family. My inheritance. My perfect place with my perfect people.

Thanks God for Answered Prayer, Jehovah Jireh.
Written October 6, 2002, 2:17 a.m.

Healing After Divorce:
Men Speak Up

"Good Man" Raphael Saadiq
"I Wanna Be Down" Brandy
"She's out of My Life" Michael Jackson
"Daddy's Home" Jermaine Jackson
"High Hopes" SOS Band

Men Have Deep Feelings

"I would have been more open with my feelings and concerns during the marriage, because that may have kept me from getting as frustrated as I did at certain points. I would have also made a more concerted effort to keep our parents out of the relationship." Mr. P

Speaking Up Helps

"Not only is it important to heal after divorce, but it's also important to heal after any type of unfavorable end to marriage or deep friendship. If you allow a negative 'vibe' to continue into a new relationship, it will likely fail. You ultimately will compare the old with the new, if you can't let go of the past. In doing so, you're not being fair to the new person.

When moving on, you must have an open mind to receiving someone new, who has nothing to do with what went wrong with the last person. It's best to cultivate and forge a new beginning by learning from and burying the past, especially, if it was toxic to you. Be prepared to love and be loved from a different platform in life." ~ H.R.

136

Why Divorce?

People get divorced for so many reasons. It's not always because of cheating, however, especially in today's world, it seems that so many men and women are stepping outside of their covenant to "get some satisfaction." That doesn't usually work.

"As men, we have to understand that the value of the woman's intellect far outweighs the attraction of greener grass outside of our yard. Our minds must prevail over our loins and our worldly desires. Most of all we must learn that real strength is being strong enough to be gentle and loving. We must submit to God before we can ask a wife to submit to us. We must Love the Lord — FIRST — and our wives as He so loved the Church. I stand strong on my words and my faith and am very happy of the man I grew into.

The toughest aspects of divorce for me were: hurting the heart of a woman I loved; being alone even though it was my choice; and facing mutual friends (of ours when we were a couple), knowing it was my fault.

I recommend that people seek spiritual counseling and look in the mirror hard and long. Think back to the reason you got married and PRAY. If I could change something, I would have become a spiritual man earlier in my life and I would do my very best to honor the words I spoke in my ceremony — treating them as a covenant between God, my wife, and myself.

I recommend that people get a clean, clear, full-sized mirror and a Bible and get to know yourself and the Lord and make sure that you are whole and complete before going back out there." ~ Tony M.

STRATEGIC PLANNING STEPS TO SOUL RESTORATION

1. **Identify the (real) cause of the divorce.** Come to terms with what happened and seek help if you need it. Don't keep your thoughts or feelings bottled up, as most long-term illnesses are stress-related.

2. **Start healing.** By acknowledging your role within the relationship and what you did or did not do to contribute to the breakdown will help you, even if it hurts at first.

3. **Forgive.** This includes your former spouse and you. The reality is, once it's over, you did the best you knew how to do.

4. **Get into spirit.** Establishing or maintaining a spiritual connection is a key to forgiveness. A journey through the Psalms in the Holy Bible is a great way to receive the Word. An ongoing process, the freedom available to you through faith and understanding will bring you clarity and wholeness.

5. **Be committed.** Be committed to learning from mistakes, trying new ways to handle things, and establishing open lines of communication with your ex if children are involved.

6. **Plan to love again.** Start with loving and appreciating you, loving you. Get back "to your fighting weight" and prepare yourself, mind, body, soul and spirit.

7. **Rejoice each day.** Each day is a new opportunity. Enjoy the gift!

Resist Temptation

You got divorced for a reason. And sure, going backward (still 'dealing' with your ex spouse in intimate ways), may seem like a logical thing to do because there would naturally be a 'level of comfort' however, if you have gone through the physical process of getting a divorce, it's unfair to your ex and to you to 'keep dipping.' It will only delay the ability to move on. And it's tough for women, especially, to separate the emotions from the realities (and finalities) of divorce. Healing matters and everyone deserves the chance to experience it.

The Children

"Before getting divorced, make sure that you have exhausted every option viable before getting divorced. If that has been done, know when to walk away and do so." ~ Mr. P

Using your kids to get back or to hold something over our heads or just making things difficult when the man is doing everything in his power to express his love and concern as a father despite the turmoil or discomfort of going through a divorce is not okay.

It is wrong when parents start using the children to manipulate or for leverage because the children are the ones who suffer. When you have a willing parent who wants to be a part of their lives, embrace that and appreciate it. Don't turn it around and abuse it or use it in a calculating way.

Parenting

There are many committed fathers who want to be consistent in the lives of their children, despite the "status" of the adult relationship with the mother. Everyone is affected by divorce in some way; no matter your role, please consider what he has to share, as you are making your moves and picking your battles. In the end, the war isn't with the children.

FATHERLY CONSIDERATIONS WHEN DEALING WITH CHILDREN AND DIVORCE

1. Deciding how custody would be arranged and the financial aspects can be difficult. Be actively involved in the arrangements and make mutual decisions about what's best for your family.

2. The finality of the divorce and the realization that the time with children will not be the same.

3. The kids didn't ask for the divorce, so do everything in your abilities to remember that fact. If the parents are able to remember that the kids are what count, they should hopefully be able to foster a respectfully amicable relationship for the children.

"We actually get along better now than we did during the last few years of the marriage.

It's alright to talk to someone. Men in general try to hold in our feelings and that leads to unnecessary stressful moments. It's also important to realize that you are not a failure. People generally don't get married to get divorced, but is happens. The key is to learn from the experience and grow as a person. You will be a better person going forward not only for the sake of a relationship, but also overall." ~ Mr. P

"Extraordinary relationships don't just happen, they are built strategically." ~ Water

(Re)-Discovery After Divorce

"It's Over" Ohio Players
"Nothing Left to Say" Mint Condition
"A Change Is Gonna Come" Leela James
"What Goes Around Comes Around" Lalah Hathaway
"Free" Will Downing

The divorce itself was the healing for me. LOL.

For me, spending alone time to rediscover myself. Doing the things I loved and pampering myself.

We hear a lot of people – not just women, talk about rediscovering... How did you lose you? What did you do to find you again?

When I got married I don't think I had truly found myself. I was still growing. The marriage was a combination of perceived obligation, pressure, and escape from other bad situations. I will skip the details of the marriage but I stayed too long after things went south...

After I left and was on my own again. I had to do a lot of forgiving of a lot of people and come to grips with reality. We cannot change people. Your parents, significant other, and your friends are who they are. I had to be who I was, not what others told or expected me to be. Also, I had to stop looking back at what I thought I should have gotten and get over the upset about what I thought I was cheated out of.

I'm just getting there – three years out of my divorce. I had to accept the responsibilities that come with my gifts and talents. ~ Ashley S.

Faith and Confidence
After Abuse

"Open up My Heart" Yolanda Adams
"Heaven Must Be Like This" Ohio Players
"Heaven Right Here on Earth" Natural Four
"Fly Like a Bird" Mariah Carey
"Sent from Heaven" Keyshia Cole

As a divorced person, I can say that there are a lot of emotions that go on. There's no set way to heal from it. It's like a death and you have to go through the phases of a death. Grief, anger, hurt, etc.

For me the first year was literally about survival. It was about just getting through daily life and finding some sense of "normalcy." I got baptized and recommitted myself to God. I found a great therapist.

After that first year I went through 34 days straight of crying. All the things I'd felt over the last year that I hadn't dealt with finally broke and came to the surface. After crying and thinking I was losing my mind, I finally had to stop and turn within, which is ultimately what brought my healing. I had to stop and look at my role in the demise of the marriage.

My ex cheated and was also emotionally, mentally, and verbally abusive. While I in NO way believe that I deserved any of that, I did have to stop and examine why I allowed myself to get involved with someone like that. The reality was that he was who he was when I married him and because I was in love with the idea of marriage and not in love with myself, he was able to be in my midst.

In my search toward self and the willingness to deal with my "stuff," and myself, I was able to find forgiveness for him. At the point that I was able to forgive him, was when I can say that my personal growth and happiness really came in to being.

While I was going through an extremely rough emotional period, my Dad told me, "You have to forgive him because as long as you don't, you give him control in your life."

*It's **not** an easy journey and it's not something I would wish on my worst enemy, but on the other side, the peace and sense of love of self that I have are something I couldn't have imagined three years ago when I was in the midst.*

I had to come to terms with me and my insecurities, issues and "stuff." I didn't realize just how much I had and how much it controlled my actions/decisions. While going through it sucked, my marriage/divorce was one of the best things that could have happened because it forced me to deal with myself. I don't know that I would have been as willing or compelled to do so on my own.

Do you know where your "stuff" came from? Did something happen when you were younger that caused you to feel like you weren't worthy of a better relationship/love/self-love?

Yes, I know where it came from!!!! In some ways I was still operating as that skinny, pimply faced, Jheri curl wearing 14-year-old girl with glasses that the boys didn't like. At least that was how I perceived the reaction. While I didn't look in the mirror and think I was unattractive, my actions said otherwise.

I was also everyone's baby in my family and their level of expectation was high in some ways. But at the same time, they would say stuff like, "Well you're the baby so you don't have to learn to do this or you don't have to try to do that." As a result, I would do things that got their attention but it was more about getting them to see that I was capable of doing things. In relationships and just life, for me, not being able to do it all was like admitting failure.

*It's taken me a **long** time to accept that I'm fine just as I am and that I don't have anything to prove to anyone. I had to start by looking at myself in the mirror every day and saying something positive. As simple as it sounds that was **really** hard for me to do in the beginning.*

Wow. I think you are very smart and very beautiful. It's interesting because I didn't know you back then. What you've said is helpful because when people look at you — all we see is confidence!

Now, what you see is confidence because I have finally accepted me as I am and I really love myself. That doesn't mean the feelings of insecurity don't crop up, but I now know what they are, and how to deal with them when they do. And again, that's exactly why I talk about it because we all have insecurities and if it helps anyone to know they aren't alone, then it's worth it. ~ Interview with Anise W.

Comments

One reason that what Anise has shared is so powerful is because it's real, raw, and true — so many people, if they read this, can begin to question themselves, their actions, and their choices — especially those who may still be in the relationship and/or the grief process...and too many times people aren't willing to admit:

1) Their role

2) The importance of counseling

3) That they need help, time, and God!

Interestingly enough, my therapist (after my own divorce) once told me that the best way to get the most out of therapy is having a spiritual base and understanding that one's spirituality or lack of it, is what can either help or hinder their mental growth. That was during my third counseling session...as a result, I went to church the very next week and the entire course of my life changed (for good) as a result. ~ Water

And Jesus said unto her
"Daughter, be of good comfort: thy faith hath made
thee whole; go in peace."
Luke 8:48

Moving On With or Without Closure

"Go on and Cry" O'Bryan
"All About Love" Earth, Wind & Fire
"Alright" Janet Jackson
"Before I Let Go" Maze featuring Frankie Beverly
"Butterflies" Floetry

How Do I Heal After Divorce?

The answer is time. Time eventually heals our wounds.

What I'd ask is, how long does it take? It can take years! Or, it can take a lot less! From experience, I know it depends on who initiates the breakup, who gets rejected. Whoever gets rejected in the breakup has the hardest time healing. So, then healing is a long drawn out process.

In my past, I initiated the breakup/divorce. For me, I believed I had no choice, given the fact that drugs played the part in my partner's life. I was no competition against the drug-addicted husband. So, breaking it off was actually a relief and a start to healing. The healing was quite different because I was relieved of all the problems associated with the life of a drug-addicted husband. Don't get me wrong, it was still hard. Now, this is what I did...

I made a written out plan about how I'd make it by myself and followed it to the "T"! I read the book, "The Language of Letting Go" by Melodie Beattie. I still read it to this day. I had kids, I had to go on, and I had to take care of them. I put my faith in God. God saw me through. Yes, I thank God! I have raised three children on my own. My daughter, first born, very determined and successful, my second born needs prayers every day, and my third is just beginning adult life and is determined to make his dreams come true.

Now Getting Back to My Point of Rejection...

In my last relationship the man whom I will always love, rejected me. To this day, I really don't have a clear reason why! All I know is that I must accept it. At this time, it has been about three months, and I still to this day think of him every minute. He meant the world to me.

I know that he's not perfect, nor I, but, I felt he just got it! We used to say that to each other "You get it!" We had such a deep connection. So when our sudden breakup happened, I couldn't believe it. I began to feel so guilty. I began to feel like "What did I do wrong?" I so believed that he was my soul mate. He was so endearing to all my family and friends, to where they loved him as much as me.

*Right now, I'm full of tears because I miss him so. He is a wonderful person that was so good to me. So generous to me and so loving to me. I thought it was unconditional! But, I was wrong. So now I am faced with **healing**. And I must say, this one will take awhile. But, I will heal. I will keep faith in myself and in God first! Relationships take so much constant work. I only want to be in a relationship with that person that will weather the storms of our imperfect selves. I wonder if I ever will!*

To me, being in a loving, lasting relationship is the most accomplishing desires of life. I am giving my healing to God and in time I will be healed. ~ Raw Expression from A.S.

The Rebound

"Sexual Healing" Marvin Gaye
"I'm Ready" Tevin Campbell
"I'm Ready" Mint Condition
"99 Problems" Jay Z
"Complicated" Rihanna

More People, More Problems

"Sometimes it can take years to be by yourself to get over the past relationship or situations. You may need a lot of time to do that. It depends on you and/or the circumstances. Please also keep in mind, and be fair to the new person and don't hold them accountable for what didn't work in the past. If you start noticing signs that happened before, maybe you just weren't ready to get involved again, at that point." ~ Ice

You are fresh from a break up and you think you are ready to entertain someone new. So you sign-up for dating sites, you wear your best outfits to the clubs, and you flirt with every decent person you see. Those are usually acts out of insecurity, not from places of confidence and this can be dangerous, hurtful, and unhealthy, leading to short-term results.

You need a time to get through the circumstances and emotions of your recent relationship before moving into something new, if your goal is for long-term love. Welcoming another person into your "sacred space" too soon may cause problems. You run the risk of creating a rebound situation.

Usually, the rebound relationship doesn't work out because someone is not really into the other person for the right reasons. Sure, having someone else to "fill in the space" can help to "get over" the last relationship however, by involving someone else in the mix, you may be asking for more fall-out. This is why healing is so important.

COMMUNICATING & COMPROMISING

IT TAKES COMMUNICATION & COMPROMISE.

To trust, create understanding, help you get along and to build your relationship takes communication & compromise.

Learning to Listen

"Listen to Your Heart" Aretha Franklin
"Crying Over Time" Alexander O'Neil
"My Funny Valentine" Chaka Khan
"Heard it All Before" Sunshine Anderson
"Stop, Look, Listen to Your Heart" The Stylistics

Sometimes the pain is so deep and hurtful that all a person can do is cry, or throw up, or yell, or breathe. Just staying alive in that moment, when it feels like giving up or giving in. Have you ever felt that way?

At those moments, when the temptation is to start to run or hurt someone else, is the very time to just listen.

What is the Message?

That you made a bad choice? That you could have said or done something better? That you deserve better than what you have? That the person that you love or who loves you is (or isn't) "the one" for you?

Whatever the situation, war often begins as an internal struggle and the battles erupt and overflow to the people in your life. If your partner is the closest to you, he or she usually gets the majority of the wrath – whether you know it or not.

Listening to the real issues, within you; the ones that are because of your relationship; and the ones that you can't control is a step to love.

What Can You Do?

You can pray. You can write down your thoughts and feelings. You can chat with your partner and genuinely listen to them – the things they say, do not say, and show. You can practice being patient and acknowledge the fear, pain, or confusion which may be holding you captive. We can't solve it here but it's a start.

Insecurities

"Pain" Ohio Players
"Love Is a Hurting Thing" Lou Rawls
"Hanging on a String" Loose Ends
"Control" Janet Jackson
"Human" Human League
"Somebody's Watching Me" Rockwell

We all have insecurities because we are human. As a result, sometimes we belittle or behave in controlling manners.

"Ego is the (false) driving force behind most of the war in our lives. Ego separates us from our real selves." ~ Water

Women, you can't belittle a man and expect him to respect himself, let alone you. Talking down to him, speaking out of turn, anything that is kind of threatening, coming from a woman, undermines his trust and confidence in you and ultimately, your relationship.

Self-Esteem Issues — the confidence levels may be low and he needs to feel support from his partner that he can handle, will provide, and fix things for his home. He needs to feel and act like a hunter — powerful and equipped to handle things for the woman and for his family. Be real and realistic.

Men, trying to control a woman will cause everyone grief. Most women who are with you want to be. They have chosen you — and are usually willing to work with you.

King of Hearts

"Your Love is King" Sade
"Is it a Crime?" Sade
"Kiss of Life" Sade
"Smooth Operator" Sade

We Love You

"Men, what you need to know is, your woman probably loves you and doesn't want to go anywhere — she just needs you — more of you — she needs to connect to your thoughts and feelings and understand what makes you tick. She may or may not be able to express this to you but, in her soul, it's probably true."
~ Water

Men have hearts, hopes, dreams, and real needs. It's easy for women to expect men to be the providers, the rocks, the initiators, and the strong arms in relationships — and many men are willing to play these roles.

So, What's Missing?

Understanding, compassion, and the building up of men.

We as women must show them how much we love and appreciate them not only in our words but also in our behavior. Emphasizing our appreciation for their opinions, input, and efforts is so important. The way we ask for things, the way we respond to things, is so crucial to the delicate balance of love and respect. Showing them that they matter to us and that we appreciate them and love them in ways that they need to be shown can be confusing because men and women are different.

At times, when we do ask them to communicate and we don't agree or like what they have said, sometimes we shut them down before they really get started. When a man is being open, take advantage of those moments and listen. Do your best to listen versus just hearing him. Listening is active. Hearing is passive. When you are just hearing, you are on autopilot or simply waiting to respond. When you are listening, you are engaged and have a much better chance of interpreting the real message.

Remember this because in their willingness to be open, communicative, and vocal about their personal needs, desires, and goals too many times they clam up because women can't see past themselves or "the family/kids."

It's not easy being a man in today's world. Make it safe (and consistent) for him to share his concerns and his *fears*. Make it easy for him to feel good about himself — whether he's gotten a raise, a promotion, lost some hair, or gained a few pounds.

Women, what you need to know is, your man has a whole different perspective about himself, you, your relationship and life in general, than you do. We're not talking about the 20 year olds or even the early 30 year olds — we're talking about grown men who have seen a lot, perhaps done a lot, and who are faced with choices each day. He needs to know that you are here with him for real — not just when he can "pay the bills."

Let's put muscles aside and focus on ways to reach the heart of a man, this one's for you guys.

Men and Space

"Travelin' Man" Masqueraders
"Midnight Train to Georgia" Gladys Knight
"Running Away" Maze featuring Frankie Beverly
"International Lover" Prince
"Getaway" Earth, Wind & Fire
"Can We Talk?" Tevin Campbell

Once you have established a firm foundation for your relationship, it's especially important to give your partner space, especially men. Sometimes they just want to get away – and it may be to the dry cleaners, the barbershop, watching a game with his friends, or to clear their heads while driving down the highway listening to their favorite music.

Ladies, it's easy to be clingy. It's tougher and smarter to be trusting and allow him to feel comfortable renewing and coming back with a renewed attitude and mind.

Men, your behavior leading up to the times you need your space will determine how your woman reacts when you request/inform her that you are taking an afternoon or evening away. Please don't act like you are taking your woman for granted and also be smart about it. Communicate with her, don't stay out until unacceptable hours, and don't make a habit or pattern of being gone at times she may need you or want you.

Couples, an occasional weekend night out with friends is okay, however, leaving your mate alone every Friday or Saturday is not okay. And if you've been known to flirt too much, been caught in the midst of bad behavior, or you are going through extremely stressful times as a couple, ask yourself if you want that space because you need it or because you are trying to avoid dealing with what's on your mind or the situations that are happening.

Freedom is in truth; always remember that.

Admitting the Truth

"Got to Be Real" Cheryl Lynn
"Your Body's Callin'" R Kelly
"Feel That You're Feeling" Maze featuring Frankie Beverly
"I Can't Get Over You" Maze featuring Frankie Beverly
"Knocks Me off My Feet" Stevie Wonder
"I Wanna Be Free" Ohio Players
"Check It Out" Tavares

If you don't tell the truth, you won't be free. If you do tell the truth, you may be set free. Telling part of the story and letting the drama unfold is just asking for trouble. Many times mates get upset about the way they find out things. Hearing things third hand, by accident, or because someone is trying to sabotage you or your relationship breeds negativity and mistrust. Things are going to happen and everyone messes up sometimes. Being accountable and admitting your role shows maturity, compassion, commitment to the relationship and respect for your mate.

"We (as men) don't operate or communicate based on emotions. We know that even though you think (as women) you can handle the truth — mentally, emotionally, and physically you will break down if you really knew what had or was happening in most cases. It's because, as men we do care, that's why it's hard to tell the whole truth because you all get so emotional. Then we think, 'You still can't handle it so I'm just going to give you a little of it.' It may not be right, but it is why some people don't tell it all." ~ Ice

"What I don't understand is, what's so hard? If we are in this relationship, what are you doing that you can't talk about? Does it mean that we shouldn't be together if you are doing so much that

you think I can' t handle it? It seems like the easy way out — for the men at least." ~ *Water*

"Nobody says it's fair, it's just a difference in the make up between men and women and that's the harsh reality, period." ~ *Ice*

"Excuse my language, but that's bullsh*t!" ~ *Water*

So, the next time you spend some extra cash on that item that you didn't need, put the cash or card away. Or, if you "find yourself" in a situation which you know you wouldn't approve of if the situation were reversed, get your butt up and leave, just say "NO!" Or, be mature enough to communicate openly about what's up. Admit the truth. See what happens. Needless war is not becoming.

Power in Forgiveness

"You're the Best Thing in My Life" Dramatics
"Free" Deniece Williams
"Ordinary People" John Legend
"If You Don't Believe" Deniece Williams
"Count on Me" Whitney Houston & Ce Ce Wynans
"Everything's Gonna Be Alright" Al Green
"Believe" Robin Thicke

Failed expectations are the primary source of conflict. Often we expect perfection but there's no such thing...the answer is forgiveness.

Forgiveness does not necessarily mean forgetting, yet if you say you have forgiven, it means letting it. In other words, you can't keep bringing up the past or punishing your partner because it could condemn the relationship.

"Forgiveness is a state of mind and a spiritual state of being. It means that for me to forgive, totally, it's not just forgiving whatever act or emotionally healing from whatever hurts, but also understanding the why, recognizing the emotional pain, and having the desire to overcome it." ~ Ice

Forgiveness and putting it in the past means we aren't bringing it back to the forefront and it continues to have an unnecessary strain on the relationship that most couples can't get past and then they get stuck. This is where constructive conversation, mediation, or even counseling may need to take place. The mediator's role is to provide fair, objective assessment of each party's version of the story or act that if not counseled, ultimately leads to a mental and emotional standoff.

In Betty Wright's song, *"No Pain, No Gain"* she gives a recipe for having a successful relationship. She describes it vividly and likens the nurturing of the relationship to a flower — needing sunlight and water. In other words, a relationship takes work. She goes further to say that the secret ingredient is forgiveness.

Power Through the Struggles

Resentment can lead to arguing, verbal jabs, fighting, poor choices, and battles, which undermine the core of your relationship and could end it. Acting as if "nothing happened" will lead to bad behavior on one of or both of your parts at some point.

Problems will happen in relationships and that's part of life. If you are unwilling to forgive, you will ultimately end up single because financial issues, stubbornness, unkept promises, broken agreements, missed appointments, lack of accountability, challenges with fidelity, being untrustworthy, or even forgetfulness could be the nails in the coffin if left unchecked.

Power Team

Decide if your relationship is important to both of you — and if it is, you must face the issues to win the war as a team. Build your strength to forgive if you are going to make it through as a couple. You must plan to succeed together.

As with any great business, worthy venture, or harmonious relationship a strategic plan must be worked. Work your plan and don't let your plan work you. In other words, you have to stay on track with your goals as you work your plan.

If you allow your plan to work you, you allow distractions, emotions, and excuses to stop you from succeeding and getting through to peace and trust.

THREE STRATEGIES TO FORGIVENESS

1. In our human form and state – nothing is guaranteed and nothing is perfect so watch where you set your bar, your expectations... be willing to compromise but just don't compromise yourself or your partner.

2. Understanding that forgiveness is an internal process. Allow your spiritual muscles to lead the way.

3. Inspect what you expect; trust but verify; and be energized through spirit, love and working together to live as a Power Couple.

POSTLUDE

MOVING FORWARD.

Preparing for Love

"You Don't Have to Hurt No More" Mint Condition
"I Got a New Attitude!" Patti LaBelle
"Ain't Leaving Without You" Jaheim
"You Don't Know My Name" Alicia Keys
"You're All I Need (To Get By)" Marvin Gaye
"Please Send Me Someone to Love" Sade
"Feel Me" Cameo
"I Found My Baby" Gap Band
"Imagination" Earth, Wind & Fire

Yes, it's important to forgive the pain, frustration, and disappointment from your previous relationship. Healing is essential because it frees space in your heart to love again or perhaps for the first time, for real.

Everyone needs time to reflect on what you want and don't want. What you can and cannot give and on how deep you will allow your love to go. It starts with self. And if you don't know where to start, get some help. Therapy does work.

Understanding your role is critical to the fresh new, committed person that you will become and be truly available in and for your new relationship(s). It's too easy to have bitter feelings and start negatively. It takes patience, loving kindness, honesty, and work to heal and to be prepared for the love relationship that you desire and ultimately deserve.

If you already had the answers, you would have what you really want so, be courageous and work on loving you first.

Life

"Life" K-Ci & JoJo
"Remember the Time" Michael Jackson
"Concentrate on You" LTD
"Happy Feelings" Maze featuring Frankie Beverly
"If Loving You is Wrong, I Don't Wanna Be Right" Luther Ingram
"Here I Stand" Usher

The four-letter word "Life" has caused us – allowed us to be here today. As we sit, whatever thoughts, feelings, attitudes, and actions we have had, have caused us to be right here – right where we are.

Are You Satisfied?

Oftentimes the answer is "no," but let's ask perhaps a better question – "What would it take to satisfy you?"… Yep, it's a tough one. Honestly though, have you taken the time to consider what thoughts, feelings, attitudes, and actions you would need to choose in order for you to be satisfied? Yep, that's a lot of work.

What Do You Really Want?

In your life? Let's break it down…In your home and relationships? Qualities you want in your mate? In your spiritual life and community? In your finances? In your health? In your work and educational endeavors? Yep, that's a lot to consider.

Why Does it Matter?

Oftentimes, as humans, we are conditioned to think, feel, and act in certain ways — based on the cultural influences in our environments from a young age... you've heard it before but, really think about it — what patterns or habits do you have that are keeping you right where you are?

Remember the Time?

Think about when you were in kindergarten, first or second grade. You were probably enthusiastic, daring, energetic, and a risk-taker... ready to raise your hand as soon as a teacher formed a question. Outgoing. Confident. Tenacious.

What Happened?

Even if you were more introverted than some, there was probably an inner knowing that pushed you to try things, explore and ask questions, until you were satisfied with the results. Yet, one day, somebody might have said, "Children should be seen and not heard." Or, "Do as I say, not as I do." Or, how about just "NO!" Yep, Life.

Please Choose!

Choose the thoughts that will put a smile on your face (your appearance will improve and so will your tone of voice!). Choose your feelings about yourself, your abilities, and your current circumstances (emotions are temporary, feelings are where you live) and reinforce them with what you actually want.

Choose your attitude — it will make you and break you. Choose your actions — with practice and a plan you can get the results you really want – with practice and with a plan you will get the results you really want... yep, "with practice and a plan, I will get the results I really want."

Are You Willing?

And if so, what are you willing to do to help define you? Let's be less complex and more transparent. Don't waste your time hiding who you are, but spend more time in allowing them to see who you really are.

Think about one thing you really want – perhaps it's confidence, patience or love... just choose one – and focus on that one word every morning seven times, and every night seven times, in your mirror for seven days, and imagine the gift your life will reveal.

Your heart is the center of love. Sometimes the internal struggles are the reason that you have so much war in your relationships. When you know this, you treat yourself better and everybody wins.

Good Men

"All True Men" Alexander O'Neil
"Coming from Where I'm From" Anthony Hamilton
"Papa Was a Rollin' Stone" The Temptations
"The First Time Ever I Saw Your Face" Roberta Flack
"Love's Theme" The Love Unlimited Orchestra
"All the Things Your Man Won't Do" Joe
"Hello" Isley Brothers

Men, it's easy to be hard, full of pride, and do the "same ole' same ole'." If you really want love – real love, harmony at home, peace, and to feel proud about who you are and what has become of your life, it takes maturity, willingness to change, and coming from your heart.

Three Simple Things to Help You and Everybody in Your Life

1. **Smile, Laughter** – because it is therapeutic to smile and it's a good start to having a good day.

2. **Resolve** – When you get down, and knocked out, are you still looking down, or are you down and looking up? If you can handle what life throws out you, and keep going after your desired outcome, it's okay. Still want to look up.

3. **Network** – Don't be afraid to reach out and to expand your horizons. Don't be afraid to venture outside of your box and always stay connected with people. The more people you know and the more people who understand you, the easier life can be.

Hope and A Bright Future

"It's Love" Jill Scott
"Right & Wrong Way" Keith Sweat
"Hope, Wish & Pray" Lina
"Hope That We Can Be Together Soon" Harold Melvin
"Black Butterfly" Deniece Williams

"As a man, know that love is not dead. Once you understand what you want and have a spiritual connection, you will find yourself reaching a place that you can only dream of. Set your goals, set your standards, create your plan and follow that plan. Stay true to yourself, stay true to your heart, live, love and learn." ~ Ice

That's what you are entitled to have and experience. Your choices will dictate if you live up to your inheritance. Too many times we let the past influence the future. Let's face it – who hasn't been hurt? Every grown person with a heart has been hurt. So, take a journey into what's causing the fear and the pain. Perhaps it is stopping you from moving forward? Putting the past behind is not easy but it is possible!

"Open your heart to possibilities, allowing the light of God to give you what you need. You can have plans however; you must allow space for surprises, delights, connections, and the time it takes for things to unfold. As Ice says, 'Building Las Vegas didn't happen overnight.' Hope comes from the head and heart, through the soul and the spirit. Don't get stuck in a 'little idea' of you, but get freedom in knowing that beyond you there is a force working to pick up the pieces in the darkest hours, the brightest days and even through confusion and healing!" ~ Water

With "A New Attitude" and some steps in the right direction, you can begin to peel back the layers and start to smile at you!

"Others take notice of your radiance. Share your happiness." ~ A Fortune Cookie

Ice Weighs In

"If This World Were Mine" Luther Vandross & Cheryl Lynn
"Solid As a Rock" Ashford & Simpson
"Forever My Lady" Jodeci
"When a Man Loves a Woman" Percy Sledge
"Piece of My Love" Guy
"Here and Now" Luther Vandross
"Never Had a Love Like This Before" Tavares

It's the end of the book and it took a lot to get here. I'm glad we've been able to share some things with you and I hope it's put some things into your toolbox to help you experience a relationship worth having.

Working with Water on this book has been intense, frustrating, sweet and good, just like our relationship. Taking the time to give her what she wants isn't always on my schedule or part of my program. Not because I don't care but because I have plans, goals, and stuff to do. Isn't that like life? A lot going on and so many expectations. I'm just telling you the truth, as I see it today so, here are some of my biggest personal challenges.

Being Totally Honest

One of my biggest challenges is being truthful – being totally honest. Why? Because the truth hurts and I've been hurt in many different ways. It kind of instilled in me to do what I can do to not hurt others. And sometimes not being so honest helps people avoid being hurt – including me.

Fatherhood

Another challenge is being a father because they (the kids) are so overexposed to things. With today's mass media opportunities and abilities, it makes it hard to parent. I often feel like I want to bottle up my children and keep them close – just to keep them safe. At the same time, I want them to see and understand what's happening in the world. They need to be able to build defense mechanisms and to rise above.

Many fathers and their kids are not talking and communicating on a daily basis, or they are simply not involved. On the other hand, if fathers are directly involved and being good influences, sometimes their peers may not be getting what they are getting, and that causes a problem. Being a teenager and being influenced by friends who don't have active, positive parents also presents more problems.

For example, I know my kids ask themselves, "Should I be as close to my parents as I am even though my friends aren't?" They have to fight through it because it's tough. That's sad, but it's true. I never thought I would see the day. I try to remain as close as possible. I want the best for them, because they deserve it.

God

Perhaps most importantly, my spiritual direction – I don't have all of the answers. I get pulled into a spiritual circle then I don't know what to do when I get there. What to do, when I'm in it is what I mean.

My spiritual direction is affected by physical and mental strains. I'm trying to understand it or tame it and it's difficult. What's difficult? Not knowing the answers concerning my future and not knowing where the journey is supposed to take me. I'm a yes, no kind of guy – I can say I'm black and white – I'm a facts kind of guy so it's bothering me because I want to know. And I'm not sure how I'm supposed to operate on faith, I just want to know and I don't so it's frustrating.

So, you may be wondering what happened with Ice and Water after you read the introduction...

Ice and Water

As "H_2O" mentioned at the beginning of this book, Ice Water was a name we called ourselves as a couple. Today, things are a bit different than when we started. I'm being real with you, from my heart, because that's what we've been doing throughout this journey with you.

Relationships aren't easy. She says I'm tough and I say she's bossy. I think I'm tough because growing up in New York took survival skills, and being a Chief in the Navy requires a certain mental fortitude. I don't really know how to be sweet. She is a kind and nice woman and she possesses all of the qualities I really want in a woman, I still smile when I think of her. Yet, she'll also say what she thinks and doesn't know how it turns me off or makes me frustrated at times.

Our relationship has been like a gift to both of us. We do have a spiritual connection. That has helped us both along the way. At the same time, I have a checklist of things that are important to me and one of the big ones is what I call "equal partnership." Because of our lifestyles, me as a career military guy and her as an entrepreneur, the way we operate our finances and decisions is different, and that's an important ingredient in my own personal strategic plan.

Just like I can't always relate to what she's talking about or sees, sometimes, it's hard for her to understand how much financial security, stability, and savings is for me. Did she tell you she has a really long checklist too?

When we met, we were both coming out of serious relationships with baggage. It was a great romance, she had me and I was "high on her." Things happened along the way and both of us did some things that weren't cool and didn't promote trust in our relationship. This was all going on as we were writing – it really is a soulful experience. Finishing this book became pressure, just like the relationship but it had to play out.

The Past, The Pressure and The Future

Hopefully this has been a learning experience for everyone. Ice needs to count on Water and Water needs to count on Ice. To really understand that analogy one would have to understand the pressure that comes with being involved in a true relationship. So we're taking time to focus on those things in our own personal strategies that need work.

What I've Learned in Our Relationship

Love, although it seems illusive sometimes, can be right there in your grasp. However, in today's society you need more than love to have a wholesome relationship. You need the understanding and the feeling that you both are evenly yoked spiritually, emotionally, physically, and financially. I have learned that communicating on a frequent basis brings a sense of sincerity, opens lines of consideration and thought. It is more so now than ever that one must be true to himself or herself. You must be able to look yourself in the mirror and know without a shadow of a doubt that you have put your best foot forward.

Relationship pressure can be stressful but when used the right way it can turn that dull jewel into a shining diamond. So remember that when you say, "I just want to be in love."
~ *Sincerely, Steven Charles Martin, Ice*

Holding On and Letting Go from H₂O

"When Love Calls (You'd Better Answer)" Atlantic Starr
"We Are One" Maze featuring Frankie Beverly
"When We Get Married" Larry Graham
"No More Drama" Mary J. Blige
"Ooh Boy" Rose Royce
"Good Times" Chic
"I'm Coming Back" Lalah Hathaway

Being Delusional

One of my biggest challenges in relationships is not letting go when it's time to let go. It's not just adult, intimate relationships; it's all my relationships. I'm not proud of it; it's just been my song, my story and my past. Have you ever heard *"Stop Cause I Really Love You,"* by Captain and Tennille? I really like that song!

When I love from "me" it's hard to separate the emotions, the feelings, the joy, the friendship, the loyalty, the spiritual, and memories from the health, the well-being, the respect, and the good treatment, which everyone deserves. That's a lot of "ands," but I'm leaving it that way for emphasis. When I've held on too long, I've ended up compromising myself, and that's not good for me or anyone else.

When I've loved someone and things don't work out, I feel loss and grief, and then I get scared — not necessarily out of fear that I won't love again, but because I had/have been accustomed to the routine — whichever routine that particular relationship afforded. Deeper than that, I just loved them.

176

Sometimes though, where I have gone wrong is that my love or me, or the way I love, may not be "right" for that person or for me. That's where clarity and understanding come into play. There are just some boundaries, which everyone has that can't be crossed. Unfortunately, if we don't have and keep those internal Geiger counters in place, things get cloudy and complicated.

Can You Relate?

I was reading an article, just in time for the ending to this book, and it talked about the correlation of depression and grief as it relates to marriage and intimate relationships. Finally, doctors are speaking what many of us (even men) have probably felt and not known to verbalize — that relationship break ups, deaths, losses do affect us – all of us. Mentally, emotionally, physically, and situationally, based on how "tied up you got" (i.e., finances, living together, marriage, kids, etc.).

So, what I can say is that if something isn't good for you spiritually, it will affect everything else and it will just play out for you depending on the way you wire and process things. I can look back and tell you beyond a shadow of a doubt that some of my "most treasured" relationships held me back and stunted my development. This happened, for me, by taking away my focus on work, getting new clients, being available to those others in my life who love and need me, and also from being with the One who is also yearning to share his life with me.

Let me clarify that last portion...being truly healed, complete, stable, and available to be with the One who knows, just like I do that we exist, for each other. Not that I have to go looking for him.

So, What Do We Take Away from This Book?

This journey into love and war has been real. It has been like a real musical drama with heroes, heroines, adventure and true, honest feelings. At the end of the day though, no matter how much strategic planning you apply, if the people aren't in their "real roles" you can be at battle, stay at war and stay in love. It depends on where you are, what you want, how much you've invested and ultimately, how much you love yourself. In the beginning we said, "Learning to love yourself is the greatest love of all," some of the very best lyrics courtesy of George Benson via Whitney Houston's heart-pumping version of the song.

Think about what you really need and deserve, and work toward that. I truly believe God knows the true desires of your heart and of mine. Even when I mess up, because I love Him, He corrects me, He rescues me, He comforts me, He keeps me sane, and He heals.

What's Next?

Global healing through *Relationships and Adult Conversations!* Let's work through it together.

~ From my head, heart, soul and spirit,
Jo Lena Johnson, Water

About Kevin B. Fleming

Kevin Fleming is a Hollywood Radio Veteran and Entertainment Industry Consultant. Kevin is a former VP for Perspective Records and spent almost 15 years as Program Director for several Los Angeles radio stations including KACE (R&B Oldies) & KRBV (The Beat/V-100) and KGFJ. He is also the Owner, Publisher and Editor of the Urban Buzz, the premiere urban radio and music industry newsletter since 2002.

Kevin's life and professional pursuits have revolved around radio broadcast management, the record business, and his love of music. A homeboy and classmate to some of Minneapolis' favorite musical sons Terry Lewis, Jimmy "Jam" Harris, Jerome Benton, Morris Day, Jellybean Johnson, Andre Cymone, Alexander O'Neal, Stokley Williams and of course, Prince…maybe it was something in the water that propelled him to live his dreams and share his talent with millions through his works.

A mentor, creative mind, and entertainment executive, Kevin's other guilty pleasure is playing golf. Kevin lives in Los Angeles with his wife of 27 years, Maria. They are the proud parents of Dylan, a student at Hampton University.

The Urban Buzz is the Premiere Urban Radio & Music Newsletter.
"Buzz Off!" Is the new blog from The Urban Buzz.
Both are distributed weekly to radio stations,
record companies and industry notables.
If you would like to subscribe, email
Editor@TheUrbanBuzz.com

About Steven Charles Martin

Chief Steven Charles Martin has served his country for over 22 years in the United States Navy. Chief Martin, as an Active Duty career recruiter, is a leader, mentor, and spokesperson for America's Navy. He enjoys helping people. His love for recruiting has provided optimal opportunities for young men and women across the nation. As a skilled communicator, trainer, and diversity spokesperson, Chief Martin has trained and developed hundreds of sailors and supported them in becoming the best that they can be in pursuing a meaningful and prosperous career in the United States Navy.

Steven is a native of Bronx, New York. A Mason who believes in community service, he's also an avid sports enthusiast. He is a die-hard NY Giants and NY Knicks fan. Steven credits his grandmother, Mildred Pearl Martin, for instilling commitment, passion, and understanding; and for showing him that life is what you make of it. Having a special relationship with his dad, Steven Charles Martin, Sr., he is grateful to his father for his mentoring, leadership, and commitment to excellence in parenting him as a son.

A father himself, Steven is blessed and proud of his two sons, Keenan and Clifton Martin.

About Jo Lena Johnson

Jo Lena Johnson provides essential leadership, communication and relationship building skills for today's world. Jo Lena lived in "The City of Angels" and spent several successful years in marketing & radio before focusing her efforts on purpose-driven work as an International Leadership Trainer & Communication Facilitator.

Previous books by Johnson include: "If You Really Want to Live, Be Extraordinary!" "If You Really Want to Be Successful, Get Connected! And, "A Light is Born! 7 Ways to Show Your Brilliance," a children's book. She is host of the weekly show, "It's Your Choice TV! with Jo Lena Johnson," where viewers get real advice, real responses and heartfelt ideas to improve and create the extraordinary in every aspect of life.

Helping people to express themselves through writing, Jo Lena is also the Publisher of Mission Possible Press, a division of Absolute Good Training & Life Skills Management, which she founded in 1998. Books to inspire, educate and develop people include works written by students, professionals and some of the countries most brilliant minds.

A member of Delta Sigma Theta Sorority, Inc., and an avid reader, she enjoys spending time with her friends, family and her mom's dog Poncho. Jo Lena's guilty pleasure is watching Reality TV shows. Her extensive and intuitive skills as a coach have helped many achieve personal, professional and teams goals. Jo Lena wears many hats and no matter what her role – publisher, trainer, or relationship strategist, she is a leader 100% of the time.

WE SPEAK…

WOULD YOU LIKE TO LISTEN?

Ice and Water are all about helping people have relationships worth having. They host the weekly show, "Relationships and Adult Conversations," airing on TotalTVNetwork.com. Tune in each week as IceWater, Steven Charles Martin and Jo Lena Johnson, share how differently men and women see love, dating and real life relationships – and what to do about it!

Steven and Jo Lena would be delighted to present to your group or organization. If you want a highly interactive, informative and fun presentation or workshop, contact them.

EMAIL IceWater@AbsoluteGood.com
WEBSITE StrategicPlanningForLoveandWar.com
FACEBOOK Strategic Planning for Love and War
TWITTER @AskIceWater

CPSIA information can be obtained at www.ICGtesting.com
Printed in the USA
LVOW122304080312

272199LV00001B/1/P

9 780985 276003